Celebrating the NEW WOMAN

in the family

Donald M. Joy

CELEBRATING THE NEW WOMAN IN THE FAMILY
Copyright © 1994 by Donald M. Joy
Published by Bristol Books

First Edition, January 1994

Unless otherwise indicated, all Scripture quotations are from the Holy Bible, New International Version © 1973, 1978 by the International Bible Society. Used by permission.

All rights reserved. Except for brief quotations embodied in critical articles and reviews, no part of this book may be used or reproduced in any manner whatsoever without written permission.

Cover design by Dan Wright

ISBN 0-917851-77-3

Printed in the United States of America

*Reformation Publishers
is glad to make available
this reprint on-demand*

Celebrating the New Woman in the Family

By Donald M. Joy

© 1994 Donald M. Joy
1994 First Printing Bristol Books

Printed On Demand 2008

All rights reserved. No part of this publication may be reproduced, stored in a retrieval system, or transmitted in any form or by any means—for example, electronic, photocopy, and recording— without the prior written permission of the publisher. The only exception is brief quotations in printed reviews.

Trade Paper
ISBN 978-1-60416-392-6

Trade Cloth
ISBN 978-1-60416-393-3

Reformation Publishers
242 University Drive
Prestonsburg KY 41653
1-800-765-2464
Fax 606-886-8222
rpublisher@aol.com

Printed and bound in the United States of America

Donald M. Joy will respond to your emails at: rodojoy@juno.com
See all of his publications and resources at www.donaldjoy.com

Dedicated to four generations of Joy women:

Celebrating Granddaughters —
Lesli
Jami
Heather

Honoring Daughters-in-Law —
Dorian
Julie

Affirming Wife —
Robbie

Saluting Mother —
Marie

To whom I owe my life and who finally trusted me with hers.

Table of Contents

1. Celebrating You! 7
    Stunning!
    My Promise!
    Growth!
    For All Young Women
    Hang On!

2. Woman! How You Have Changed! 15
    Fantastic Genes
    From Girl to Woman
    Behold the New Shape!
    Check the Face and Skin
    Height, Weight and Emotions
    Peace and Discipline, Now!

3. Check Those Roots! 27
    "High Investment" Parents
    High Value Daughter
    Fantastic Dad
    Maximum Mother
    Dads and Moms Together
    Brothers
    Sisters
    Family

4. Dreams Do Come True! 37
    Here's Your Dream License
    Young Women Who Speak Out
    Hang On to Your Self!
    Take Your Feelings Seriously!
    Going for Your Dream

5. Getting to Know Each Other—in Private, Slowly 45
    The Mystery of Bonding
    Father Absence and Bonding
    Crazy Bonding
    Healthy Bonding
    Entry Gate to the Pair Bond
    Foundations for the Pair Bond
    Commit or Break Up Now!

6. The Couple's Private Agenda: Consumating the Bond 57
   For a Lifetime?
   The Pair Bond's Interior Mansion
   The Citadel Chamber: Ultimate Safety
   Risk Proofing Your Marriage

7. Your Center of Gravity! 67
   Fertility
   "What Are Little Girls Made Of?"
   Sexual Pleasure
   Responsible for Pleasure
   The Female Mind
   Stand Tall!

8. Coming Back When Things Go Wrong 79
   Dealing with Abuse and Loss
   When Childhood Is Filled with Pain
   Counting Up the Losses
   Filling the Cup of Self-Esteekm
   Seduction on a summer Afternoon
   Sanctifying Sexual Energy
   Recovering from Sexual Addiction
   Caught in the Family Nest
   How Victims Survive
   Dancing with a Domineering Stressor
   Escaping Crazymaking
   When Victims Marry
   The Bottom Line

9. Take Your Curiosity to the Bible 97
   Creation and the "Image of God"
   Man and Woman as "One Flesh, Naked and Unashamed"!
   Intimate "Knowing," Intercourse, Conception and Birth
   The Taboos: Adulterating, Fornicating, and Raping
   Song of Solomon: Images of Sexual Loving
   Jesus: Ultimate Respect for Human Sexuality
   Divorce: Unspeakable Loss and Pain
   The Ghost of Lost Love
   Transformation of Failure and Loss
   Brides, Grooms, Weddings, and Intimacy

Index 113

Chapter One

Celebrating You!

We came to the University of Kentucky Hospital, dropping everything to see you. Mike and Dorian, your parents, were still in the hallway outside the delivery room. Your mother was sitting up cross-legged. I wanted to cry out *Lie down! Don't you know you shouldn't be sitting up laughing?* But she laughed anyway and bubbled up your name: "Oh! Mike! Go see if you can get Heather so they can see her!"

See her! I thought, *If this is any kind of a hospital we can't see her, and they won't give her to her dad!* But here he came rounding the corner in his green hospital scrub suit — beaming all over and cuddling you to show you off.

And there you were: Naked, streaked with a little mark of blood, the *lanugo* hair swirling all over your beautiful body, eyes wide open! I was shocked at the amazing hospital policy. But this UK teaching hospital was light years ahead of the rest of us when you were born. They were giving us some bonus "birth bonding time" with you. Three years later I would hear about birth bonding and teach it in my human development classes. But we lived it with you. Now the experts recommend "more than 15 minutes of skin, eye, and voice contact within the first two and one-half hours of life," if you want a peaceable, bonded relationship with your child!

But when you were born, I was inhibited, worried that you were in danger of being exposed to terrible things from your parents and grandparents. Nothing like that entered Robbie's head, however. Grandma took you into her arms and hung on for dear life. You examined her face in magnificent detail. She cooed and talked to you non-stop, extraverted wonder that she is. And you were the most active, intelligent human newborn I had ever seen — the only one I had ever seen, in fact! I was amazed at how attached you were to Grandma's face, how attentive to her voice. You were practically speaking to her with the high voltage intention of your face. It is not surprising that there is still a special tie between the two of you.

Stunning!

Now I watch you, Heather, at 16 and hold my breath. Jami, your cousin, and Lesli, your sister, and you are the new Joy women! Robbie and I see you almost every week. We create last minute visits to White Mountain Creamery for bedtime dessert, grab you for a Bob Evans breakfast or stop at a Wendy's Superbar on the way to Wednesday night kid's club. We can't get enough time with you to celebrate your new and wonderful entry into the adult world. We've watched you from birth to full adult height and development in a wonderful panorama of celebrations and rejoicing.

So, there goes Lesli kicking the winning point in a LYSA shootout! Jami plunges from the edge of the pool in a championship run of the summer swim competition! Heather saves the championship soccer game for her Lafayette High School team by her expert "keeper" work and captures the attention of Olympic scouts! And one by one we've gotten the signal that you were being baptized, starring in the touring church musical and welcoming us to the "homecoming concert." You are our new women in the Joy clan! I hold my breath every time I see one or all of you.

Two kinds of thoughts surge through me: *Stunning women. We've produced the best of the twenty-first century!* This thankful and ecstatic celebration is sometimes followed by a prayer: *God, Help them to give their beauty and their gracious and vulnerable lives into absolute obedience to Jesus!*

My Promise!

When I look at you, filling out your gorgeous destiny as beautiful women, dreaming your dreams of careers, of love and marriage and families, I feel connected to the next century — through you. If you return the compliment, I suppose when you look at your grandma

Chapter One: Celebrating You!

and me with our marks of ripening age, you feel anchored in the past.

I am eager for your life to be full and rich and free. So I am going to set down here all of the "trade secrets" I know about being a mature woman and living fully. Robbie, Julie and Dorian have helped to shape this book. And, as you know, most of what I know about girls and women is what I learned before I was 15 — from my mother. She is a favorite of yours and you show it week after week. At 86 she is in the best of care when you hug her and energize her days with phone calls and visits. My mother — Marie Royer Joy — had never studied human growth and development and did not have the advantage of great libraries and modern information centers. Yet she lived in transparent honesty with me. As far back as I can remember, she was urging me to make decisions of my own and giving me answers to the urgent questions I had courage enough to ask. My parents and grandparents never controlled me as a way of showing their power over me, and they did not hide their life secrets from me, either.

I am putting my best secrets in written words for you for two reasons: First, because there are so many of them — too many for a speech. Second, because I want you to be able to re-read them, weigh them and decide what to do about the issues in your own life, without having to talk back to me. I respect you so much that I want you to sort and sift out the ideas. You have already shown me that you can make tough decisions and make them well. So I know that you will be able to shake down what is here, too, and to keep the parts that are true and right for all generations.

Some of what I am writing is very personal. Yet those secrets may be the most urgent ones for you. I have taught everything I am writing here, and some people have come back 20 years later to thank me for "being there with the right stuff" when they needed it. After you've read my best secrets unveiled here for you, you can know that your Grandmother Robbie and I are ready to talk with you anytime about these or any other things that are important to you.

After I had unveiled a lot of my life secrets at a men and boys' breakfast in Toronto a few years ago, the oldest man there — older than I am — slowly got to his feet when I offered to respond to questions.

"I have a question for you," he said. I thought I might have offended him.

"Where were you when I was 15?" he asked.

Sometimes it is hard to find out the really big secrets we need to know in life. A 19-year-old college sophomore in Pennsylvania told me after a session on "pair bonding" that it was the information she needed when she was in middle school: "I grew up in the church. I always hoped something like what you just taught us was true, but nobody at home or at church ever assured me that my dream was on target. If only once I had heard what you just shared with us, I would not have had an abortion at 16."

Since most of my seminars and lectures are far from where you live, you are not likely to slip in where I am teaching. That's another reason I have written the urgent secrets here for you! You don't have to travel or register for a Rocky Mountain youth seminar to hear me talk.

Growth!

When Jason, our firstborn grandkid and your cousin, turned five, Heather, you stretched to the full stature of your three-year-old aspirations and announced, "I'll be five in a minute." And you were. We've watched all of you from birth to maturity and it seems like only a couple of those "minutes" all together.

At about five, six and seven, the three of you gave Robbie and me a wonderful Saturday's entertainment. There you came out of our play attic — the second floor storage room with its collection of antique trunks, old shoes, hats and dresses. You chose "dress up" shoes. But since it was a summer day and too hot for the heavier clothing, you stuck with your children's sun dresses. Big wads of toilet tissue expanded your busts — you giggled, calling them "boobs" — to mimic the grown-up bodies you wanted so much.

We watched the parade of "little women" for a half hour or so as you hid behind your thin masks of giggles and clomped in and out of the house. We were working in the yard, so we got a full revue as you came out of the back door. Then Jami took a spill on the sidewalk and came up crying. The sting of the concrete had left patches of missing skin below each knee. "Little women," it turned out, don't see the ground well enough to walk safely when they have overstuffed sun dresses!

But now the grace and maturity you present is real. And you not only walk safely. You have the bearing of a royal queen — confident and able to accept your place in the world of the good and the whole people who know who they are, where they came from and where they are going.

For All Young Women

I am writing not only for you, but for all girls who are bursting through into their full womanhood. You remind me of the urgent questions I had as I was hitting my teens. I am also writing this book for dozens of young women who have backpacked with my students and me in our "discipleship development through trail camping" adventures in the Daniel Boone National Forest in more than 20 trips since 1977. For all young women eager to embrace life and to achieve their highest dreams, I offer this book. Check the table of contents for the outline of each chapter. You can begin anywhere and the ideas will make sense. I wrote it "straight through" mostly, so it may read best that way. But let your real questions dictate what you search for first. As these brief chapters unfold, I will offer you the best information I have.

If you feel like a victim of abuse or feel pretty hopeless about anything, turn to Chapter 8 now. I've called that chapter full of hope "Coming Back When Things Go Wrong."

If you read straight through, here are the issues discussed in each chapter:

1. *Reflections about your value and the uniqueness I see in you.* In this chapter I have saluted you. I not only admire you in every way, but I think I would lay down my life to shield you from anything that could hurt you in any way.

2. *Ways of affirming your growth into womanhood.* You are walking right into issues of "female identity," "female roles" and "adult responsibility." You are ready for all of them, so I will describe each one so you can see it as if it were a mirror on your wall. You have everything you need to travel safely into full adult responsibility. But not all girls do, so I want your journey to be a blessing and not a tragedy. That is why I want to give you a walking tour through some of the choices you will face. And that's why I will describe some of the feelings that come with the territory of your new womanhood.

3. *How to treasure your own family — examining your "roots" as you reach out to become your own person.* You will be making good choices about your future family and ways to build quality into your own children's lives.
4. *How to "go for the gold" in setting your goals for being a responsible and trustworthy person.* This is especially important since some people have other plans for you — wanting to use you or to drag you into very destructive things.
5. *A picture of your dream of what you are and want to become as a woman.* This painting is true of every healthy girl as she embraces her new adult status. And since you are the prize of such females in the human species, I'm pretty confident I will hit the target. Give yourself permission to add notes in the margin about specifics that I don't know about.
6. *A list of decisions that will open doors and close out whole universes.* Some people worry that the biggest decisions anyone makes are those that come between 15 and 25. But I will be writing a license for you to act on your responsibility well, to use the clear imagination and reality base that you are already using and to go for it! If you can describe who you want to become and what you want to achieve, then I'll offer some strategies for turning those dreams into reality.
7. *How to manage what one of my professors once called a female "global-process sex system."* I am calling your sexual energy the "center of gravity" for your lifetime. That title suggests something about the central importance of your reproductive system to your identity, about its high energy and about its inescapable splendor. But I also want to name some of the risks to women of all ages who do not respect the power of their sexuality and keep it nicely managed. Your sexual energy can be nurtured and managed and released in wonderfully constructive ways.

The first thing Dr. Max Crocker said about you, preserved on your dad's videotape, is "It's a girl!" And in between, the most important identification you have ever worn is your female identity. As you take responsibility for your womanhood, I will tell you all I know about managing your "global center of gravity" and rising to full responsibility and pleasure as a woman.

8. *How to deal with trouble or failure.* I wrote a chapter I hope you never need to read. I've called it "Coming Back When Things Go Wrong." On second thought, you may need to read it, because with your kind of open and honest face, somebody is going to confide their tragic story by telling it to you. Your friends who trust you enough to tell you the trouble they are in may be desperate enough to give up on everybody and even on life. So the chapter can be your "good news" for people who are in pain or trouble. And you need to know, yourself, what the bottom line is if you ever feel like giving up. Since you live, along with me, in a crazy world where terrorists, mad bombers and Pied Pipers of the worst sort are working the crowds, I have closed Chapter 8 with the "bottom line." I will tell you where I stand with you if the going gets tough, or worse. I am for you — unconditionally! I urge teens in pain to begin with Chapter 8 and see that there is life after tragedy, pain, and failure.

9. *What the Bible says about all the questions you thought nobody would ever let you ask.* Since you, like I, have found Jesus calling you to the best kind of life, I've put together a chapter which offers a walking tour of what the Bible has to say about sexual things. If anybody ever suggests to you that the Judeo-Christian Scriptures are "negative" about human sexuality or the vision of becoming fully alive and human, they haven't seen the material I've pulled together for you here. Grab your own Bible as you read Chapter 9. You can locate everything I have quoted. Check out what comes before and after the parts that spoke personally to you or that made you really curious.

Lesli, Jami and Heather, I always belong to you, and you can always find me. For the benefit of other young women, I'll publish my phone number at the end of Chapter 8 — the chapter dealing with pain and trouble. I am eager to hear from anybody who needs encouragement to pick up the pieces and get on with the whole and healthy good life.

Hang On!

So that's the promise and the list of issues. Take your time, and write your questions in the margins. This is a personal book beamed into your life at a time when you deserve the privacy of a locked room, information that opens life's best secrets and permission to ask all of your questions in a safe place. Insist on getting answers you can trust.

Chapter Two

Woman! How You Have Changed!

There you were with your school friends. Your Grandma and I spotted you in Turfland Mall after school. I had read about "mall rats," but hadn't thought about having any in our family. The three of you were so at ease, so beautiful — full-grown women! We recognized Anna as you turned toward us. Then you introduced us to Cara. We had known Anna since her parents brought her home one Easter afternoon, adopting her within hours of her birth.

Exotic and different from each other as the three of you were, there was a sort of "same culture" mark on all of you. It was something about how your hair was styled and how you had chosen your clothing. It may have been in your way of walking and consuming time in the leisurely happy stroll through the mall.

"Are you shopping?" I asked.

"Just hanging out," you said. "We almost always do this after school. It's sort of on our way home. A lot of our friends are here."

Robbie and I were joining the early dinner generation for an evening meal in our favorite restaurant. As you walked away Robbie and I gazed at the three of you for a couple of minutes. The mall is full of your friends, of course, and interesting stores.

Window shopping, I thought.

Then, I noticed that Anna had stopped briefly; she was looking in a window but adjusting her hair. Windows, it turns out, are mirrors, too. The mall is a mile of mirrors and you can check your new look — your new womanhood — simply by looking in any direction and beholding your walk, your gestures, your smiles and other body language. You can monitor this new woman we admire so much. I suppose you are "growing accustomed to her face, her smile, her ways." No wonder you always look just right. You rehearse here for a couple of hours after school every day. It hardly crossed my mind that your whole reason for wanting to look just right is because the one wonderful guy in the whole universe may be looking your way.

Fantastic Genes

We wondered, of course, when you were a newborn what this girl child would grow up to be. I saw my own mother's profile in you before you were three. But you are a combination of another half-universe of wonderful genes I don't know so well. Today, what you see in the store window and what I admire when I see you is a unique woman who blends together the heritage of a thousand generations of two good sets of family ancestors. So you are a surprise package and we are watching eagerly — like children on Christmas morning — to see what is in the package.

Anna's parents must have thought about the arrival of this time of life when they asked their attorney to interview her birth mother and father "on camera." That thoughtful attorney had his wife shoot the now famous "home video" that Anna has watched a hundred times or more. The parents were young and frightened. Even in the grief of giving her up, they remained beautiful in the prime of bright and shining youth. Anna had shown us the video herself when she was about ten.

"I'm ten, and Linda was sixteen when I was born. That means she is twenty-six now. Billy was sixteen, too." *Amazing!* I had thought, *Anna calls her birth parents casually by their first names, as if they are her peers, her friends.*

Anna was lucky, having the color video images to give her an idea about the ancestral genes she carries. They were indeed beautiful young parents, and they chose life for Anna even though they could not manage to give her the home she needed.

At fourteen, Anna sat in my office telling me how lucky she is to have parents who have loved and launched her through childhood and who are the most heroic people she knows. "If anybody could pick their home, they get the blue ribbon. They are my Mom and Dad. No contest!" she reflected.

But she went on. "When I look in the mirror, I have to be thankful to Linda and Billy. They provided the raw material, and it's pretty good. Maybe I have the best of two worlds.

"I can't imagine having to make the decisions they made. I wonder if they 'got old' overnight making choices about the pregnancy and deciding what to do with me. It kind of makes me 'old' just thinking about all the trouble I caused them." Anna named two other couples who panicked and didn't let the baby live.

"Linda and Billy had to be really good folks."

Then, looking out the window, she touched her eyes with the corner of a folded wedge of tissue.

Anna is healthy, I mused as she had talked. I told her that she is a beautiful and gracious woman. And she is doing good work with her grieving and asking the right questions.

"Do you pray for Linda and Billy?" I asked Anna then. She nodded. "How do you pray?"

"Mostly I worry about them and wonder if they married each other, so I ask God to be good to them and to give them what they want. And I have such mixed feelings, so I beg God to let me find them again. Is that natural?"

"Of course. You have good instincts," I encouraged her. "Most of us have mixed feelings and don't know what to pray or what to ask for. But there are two kinds of prayers that are always right: prayers from a thankful heart and hope for other's lives to come together into God's perfect will.

"Try listing some things you are thankful for: their willingness to suffer and their wisdom in making good decisions for you, for example. Then wrap up your prayers for them with words of hope. It can include things like this: Wherever they are, together or apart, let the magnet of your love keep making them into your kind of people — always just, always kind, always ready to protect the helpless and be your agents in the world."

Adopted kids are not the only ones who worry about their genes — who they look like, what they are "carrying" in their fertility. It's a good thing for you and everybody else to look for the best stuff you can see in yourself and to bless the day you were conceived. Celebrate your genes and offer prayers of thanksgiving to God that you were lucky enough to be born exactly who you are.

Before you made that sudden transition from girl to woman, there were the carefree years when you didn't even know you had a body. "Genes" sounded to you like something you would wear. Surprise! Genes are what you wear visibly all over!

You protested when I had to brush your hair to bring you to a basic civilized look after a night in your favorite sleeping bag in our family room. You thought brushing teeth and taking baths were terrible ways to invest the scarce time in your early years.

By the time you were turning 11, I became aware we were dealing with somebody else! The *new woman* was on her way. The fancy little girl dresses were evidently sliding to the back of your closet and we were seeing a distinctly different look.

From Girl to Woman

When you are no longer a little girl, what are you? Most of the time you hear me refer to you and your friends as "women." I do that because it is the best and noblest word to describe any human being gifted with femaleness. You are a teenager now. Sometimes people refer to you as an adolescent or talk about your going into pubescence. But those are technical words and don't make good names for people.

Puberty refers to the biological changes which mark your transition from child to adult. You literally get a new body, a new look, new hair scattered over your body in very adult places and the arrival of your fertility — your sexual ripening.

Young women hit fertility on the average at age 12. You could say that a girl becomes a woman when her uterus begins to collect the nutrients that would help a baby grow. In cycles of about a month, she will have the bleeding menstrual periods. During the menstrual period you will have a few days of bleeding from the vaginal tract.

"I thought I was dying," one of my students wrote in her journal. "I was doubling over with pains and stole away to the bathroom. I was only eight years old and my mother hadn't thought to tell me about the bleeding. It took an hour or so for her and my aunt Betty to get me calmed down." The bleeding sometimes comes with pains or cramps that feel like you have been punched hard in the stomach. What is happening is that the uterus has to let go of the basic nutrients it has stored to make a baby. So when no baby is conceived during that month, the stored materials have to be flushed away to start collecting again for the next month. This "flushing out" is painful.

Ovulation sometimes begins with first menstruation, but more often comes several months later. It is the real fertility sign — the monthly release of an ovum or an egg which contains the beginning formula for creating a new person. I'll talk more about it in Chapter 7, where I describe the marvelous biology of a woman's reproduction.

Pubescence is a word built on *puberty* which refers to the two-year period extending from the time you began your wonderful growth spurt and transformation from child to adult, up through the time you gained your full height and are sexually ripened, capable of adult reproduction. Pubescence has ended when you have filled out with rounded hips and womanly breasts. Near the end of pubescence you will get an idea of how much body hair will show up. There will be a wedge of groin hair and patches of under-arm hair. Most women develop some hair on the legs and a few will notice an increase of facial hair — some pigmentation of the normal "fuzz" that is standard equipment on all children of both sexes. When it disappears, the hair follicle pattern is replaced with an almost invisible pattern of hair on the arms and legs. In males this hair takes on color at pubescence, but is not always noticeable in the adult female.

Teenager and *adolescent* are something else! Adolescence refers to the gap between the time when you are fully grown and biologically mature, and the time that the whole world respects you as the adult you already knew you were. So adolescence is something your culture creates — like a holding tank where it keeps you until you are allowed to embrace your full destiny as a woman: entering your vocation as a professional, a wife and a mother. Teenager, on the other hand, is a subculture created by creative young adults who know they are no longer children. Since nobody takes them seriously as responsible and capable adults, they "baptize" each other, and adults pick up this code word. "Teenager" designates powerless people who have to postpone real life for about ten years.

Behold the New Shape!

Young boys and girls have identical shapes. A boy and a girl wearing identical clothing and with hair of medium length are almost impossible to tell apart by gender. Not until pubescence does its two-year remodeling job can the male and female bodies be differentiated. The most visible body changes in girls are the rounding out of the hips and the expanding of the breasts.

When my sister, Anice, was turning 12 or so, she was struggling to get used to her new shape. The only full length mirror in the house was near the front door — for the final check on appearances as we left the house, I guess.

One evening, in the few minutes while we were waiting in the next room to be seated for supper, Anice preened in front of that long mirror, stroking her hips. Coming from her bedroom, our Grandma Royer, then nearing 80, walked up behind Anice, unconsciously mimicking Anice's "side-stroking" gestures.

"These hips!" Anice muttered. "I don't know what I am going to do with these hips!"

"Hips?" Grandma Royer said, only a couple of feet behind Anice, stroking her barrel-like sides. "I don't have any hips."

The scenario is permanently filed in Joy household family humor, as you can imagine. But we had all seen pictures of a 20-year-old beauty named Mary Francis Moyer in the days when David Aquilla Royer was beginning to squire her around. They were mere neighborhood children when Lincoln was shot. But when they entered the 1890s, they were as firm and shapely a young couple as any of us could be.

If Grandma Royer had done watercise or gymnasium aerobics, her hips might have held their tone, as yours will. Women who are in rigorous athletic training often get their fertility cycle later than those who simply keep in good condition or do not exercise at all. And women who are extremely active athletically, especially the runners, often loose their fertile cycle all together until they become less active. Grandma Royer was a farm woman, active with heavy duty work, but not careful to watch her diet and exercise to keep her womanly shape.

So enjoy your new shape. The hips carry the major supply of fatty tissues in which you are beginning to store your unique female hormones — the estrogens and related chemicals that charge your fertility. I'll talk more later about the reproductive system, but you'll be glad to know that a young girl's first menstrual period seems to be more related to the "height and weight" charts than to age. She needs a thickening of the body compared to height in order to be "charged" with her fertility.

Chapter Two: Woman! How You Have Changed! 21

But it is the breasts that will drive you crazy one way or another. There is evidently nothing to make you more self-conscious than to have a sudden ballooning of your bust until you neither look nor feel like the little girl you recently were. Conversely, there is nothing more painful, many women have told me, than to be "flat chested" into your late teens and 20s. The underdeveloped girl also dies a thousand deaths of embarrassment. These under-breasted girls are almost always the "under-weight" girls or women, too, compared to height. The American dream girl who is skinny and full breasted is an unfortunate idol. Almost always these large breasted, thin hipped sex symbols are artificially inflated with surgical implants.

Check the Face and Skin

The shape of your face changes as you hit pubescence. Bone structure in both girls and boys shifts. Boys' faces tend to move cheek bones up and forward, while girls' faces tend to become more rounded, almost mirroring the reshaping of the hips.

As you discovered your face, you became suddenly aware that you were beautiful — or had the possibility. You experimented with ways to style your hair. But all the while you were studying your new facial features: eyes, eyebrows, the stunning line from temple to chin — the formation of a lovely and distinguished profile. You couldn't get enough mirror angles to satisfy your curiosity about how much you were changing. You huddled with friends you trusted. You experimented with makeup and hair styles in the safety of a Saturday marathon — far enough from Sunday and Monday to recover and get yourself back to "natural" and "comfortable" new looks. Eventually you got the right coaching about how to highlight your best features without painting everything with makeup.

Women bless us all by taking care of themselves and creating beauty in their appearance. But it is easy to fall into the "self-idol" trap. Melanie, one of my students who is strikingly beautiful, told how her mother suggested that she set a timer in the bathroom to record how many minutes each morning she spent getting pretty. "Then," her mother suggested, "spend an equal amount of time during that day in quiet reflection, Bible reading and prayer. This will be working on the 'interior beauty' that lasts forever. You won't always have a young and beautiful body. But the real Melanie will inhabit eternity."

About the time you were discovering your face in the mirror and beginning to suspect that other people were staring at you, you may have been unlucky enough to develop skin blemishes. Acne, pimples, "zits," are the curse of growing up for many people. Your whole body is a chemical laboratory exploding during pubescence. If you are struggling with the changes, sometimes you feel like wearing a sign that says, "Closed for renovation!"

Pubescence — this two-year period — often feels like a disaster zone. But look at it this way: *It is worth waiting to get this new improved body.* So talk to yourself in the mirror and thank God for the changes. You will like the finished product, even though there may be some days when you think you don't look so good. The chemical side effects which show up in skin blemishes are actually signals that your whole body is being transformed. If you like the idea of becoming a woman with all of the rights and responsibilities that go with it, then celebrate the pubescence time of transformation too.

Choose your soap carefully. Women study cleansing agents to find the exact skin care that keeps them comfortable and keeps skin smooth and soft. If your mother isn't ready to coach you here, pick out an aunt or a friend's mom who seems to be at ease and competent about these things.

When you hit your first menstrual period, you will want to get smart, too, about how to control the odors which come when the uterus empties. If all else fails, ask some gentle and good woman or phone your family doctor's office and ask for the basic tips. Physicians often have booklets which have put into print what might be embarrassing for you to ask or to talk about.

Watch your teeth, too. By now most of your baby teeth are gone. You may even get wisdom teeth behind your heavy duty molars by the time you finish high school. Or those wisdom teeth may have to come out. That is no fun, but most of us don't have much luck keeping them. Check the straightness and evenness of your teeth and the alignment where they bite together. Your dentist can coach you on how to brush to keep them clean without damaging the thin porcelain coating that you want to last a lifetime. If you have overcrowded or otherwise crooked teeth, this is the time of life to get them fixed. An orthodontist can work miracles, even with an adult with irregular teeth. But the early teen years are the very best. The "Closed for Renovation!" sign is one that a lot of teens

Chapter Two: Woman! How You Have Changed!

wear during these school years while they get their teeth lined up. But you may feel that having braces is really the in thing, so brush, polish and smile. Dazzle us all with the mouth appliances for a few months.

Use some common sense, though, and see if you can develop some habits which would correct mouth structure and straighten teeth. If you were to spend an hour a day, for example, playing a horn with a large, circular mouthpiece, you could correct many irregular alignment problems. So if you ever thought of playing an instrument, start with a trombone, baritone, trumpet or tuba. The large circular mouthpieces of these instruments press against your entire dental area. At the same time, you are pushing with air pressure behind the teeth. The combination is just right to reshape your mouth into the best of all dental displays! And you will learn how to read music and play with an impressive group. The beautiful teeth come free. Your gums are very flexible during your teen years and can be reshaped easily. Stay away from clarinet or saxophone if you already have an overbite. The reed mouthpiece will put pressure under the upper teeth, pulling them even further forward and complicating problems you may be trying to correct.

Height, Weight and Emotions

You will feel the advantage of being a woman when you hit sixth grade, or before. Girls, in general, get their full height and come into pubescence a full year ahead of boys, as a group. Boys get charged with such a heavy-duty load of hormones during fetal development that they tend to be longer in the womb and to be slower in development, in every way. So you will tend to be taller and heavier and to think more maturely than many boys at this time. You may be more easily hurt, for example, because you take yourself and other people more seriously than you did when you were a little kid. This emotional yo-yo is likely to hit you during your premenstrual days, and the menstruating week is no fun either. You may be giggling your head off one minute and feel like bursting into tears the next.

But you will stand tall and be fully developed while all those little boys are just starting their adventure into the stratosphere. Your fifth grade school class picture may be the last time until about age 21 that you can see the whole group in proportion. And there will be some amazing surprises. Boys who were "shrimps" in sixth grade may turn out to be almost seven-foot-tall giants during the college years. Many boys are still growing when they graduate from high school.

It is a fairly reliable rule that a girl almost never grows more than one inch in height after her first menstrual period. The exceptions will have something to do with that weight-height combination. And most girls will experience thickening and weight gain that may worry them as they get their full growth and their fertility. But if we can shove aside the mythology that says skinny women are beautiful, you can take pleasure in your new healthy body and go for a new wardrobe that enhances your natural beauty and your newly emerging true shape.

Peace and Discipline, Now!

If I could give you one gift about your new body it would be to give you this license: Look in the mirror and give yourself permission to be thankful for the new you. But if you could give yourself one gift that will enhance your whole life, do this: Promise that woman in the mirror that you will take care of her, feed her right, get good medical attention and be a woman full of integrity in all of her relationships — with parents, family, friends and that potential future husband and family God may give you in his time. And follow Melanie's secret formula for being a healthy and good woman:

> For every minute looking at myself in the mirror
> I spend one minute looking into the face of God
> through prayer, meditation and Bible reading.
> Exterior attractiveness deserves interior integrity.

With breasts that make you feel both wonderfully feminine and hopelessly clumsy on the basketball court, you may be tempted to retire from your favorite carefree activities. So be sure to get comfortable with clothing that supports you well, and keep a calendar on that cycle that does inhibit you a little for a few days. You can probably use an insertable sanitary product that is less troublesome than external ones for your athletic routine. Make it a point to regularly enjoy some activities that keep your muscle tone tight and your body pumping positive brain chemicals — a sort of natural high that comes from feeling good about yourself. Here are some tips:

1. Jump at the opportunity to walk instead of riding in a car if the distance to school or work is reasonable — up to a couple of miles. This gives you a workout in slow motion twice a day, and pumps you full of oxygen and keeps your heart toned.
2. Avoid elevators and escalators if you can take the stairs, even though you need to make the trip several times a day. I notice where I work that the trim folks take the stairs and the overweight stand in line to ride the elevator. Watch who you are hanging out with when the choice comes.
3. Get intentional about recreational activity. Join a church team in softball, tennis or aerobics, for example. And do the same about competitive activities if that is your cup of tea. Don't get locked into passivity. Be the active woman you honestly need to be, and juggle your family and life priorities to be a good manager of your non-renewable gift: your healthy body. Look into swimming, gymnastics, skating, field hockey or biking. Or combine them with running and enter local marathons and be a triathlete. Many of these healthy activities are part of your elective curriculum during the school years:

   Team events. If you sign up for contact sports, you are also buying a deal for building your body, watching your diet and moving with a crowd of people also committed to excellence in training and in the cooperation needed to play and win by the rules. If the sports folks at your school don't have this kind of integrity reputation, you have a problem with your school administrative and coaching staff. If you are serious about discipline and excellence, consider church, community or volunteer leagues which have the top reputation for developing positive people.

   In all team events, you are building physical skills as well as social skills. "Team players" tend to be very productive in adult careers of all kinds, and they tend to take people seriously. That makes for good performance anywhere.

   Don't overlook other team opportunities that may be more your style: debate, drama, orchestra, band and choir. These are less rigorous in physical training than contact sports, but they often require intense mental skill development, a sense of rhythm and tonal precision. The benefits are life-long and may continue as recreation and practice long beyond the adult days of touch football. Music and speech skills, for example, tend to last for a lifetime. And any group event skill may eventually turn you into a coach, a minister or a director, and your career spans much of your lifetime.

Individual events. Jump at the chance to compete against yourself as you train for piano, triathalon, cross country, golf, tennis, singing, playing, skiing, skating or swimming. While you may be part of a team for some of these in major events, the discipline is mostly individual, and your competition is against the clock or the judge's pencil. You are stretching for excellence in a field in which you are fully responsible for the outcome.

The benefits of individual events are mostly personal. You have a sense of who you really are, what you can do, and how far you can go. You may turn pro and continue an adult career after the Olympic competition you dream of. And when you scan the list, you will see that these are activities you can enjoy for a lifetime, even if you do not turn professional and make your career out of the training and skills of your youth.

I am urging you to get involved for two reasons: You need to overcome inhibition about physical activity after your body begins to change suddenly. Many girls become so passive that they put on flabby weight that is not their true or best self, but is layered on and mixed with depression and self-consciousness. But the second reason is equally as important: You have wonderful energy and time now that will be harder to find when you are finishing high school or are off to college. Many people hit college and wish they were good at something, but the hours of training are much harder to chip out of a college day or your coming adult career than out of any day of your life during elementary, middle or high school years.

So, welcome to the world of your womanhood! I am eager to help you and your family virtually abolish adolescence. Stretch to the new responsibilities that come to you as a young woman, and give your parents a chance to trust you with more and more responsibility. It looks good on you!

Chapter Three

Check Those Roots!

"How does he manage to always be here?" you asked as you watched your dad roll up in the family car at a four o'clock junior varsity event. The other man with him, it turned out, was a business contact from out of state. They had an hour and a half before dinner so your father brought his guest to the sidelines to watch you and your team.

Your parents were always there for you. And when Lesli's select soccer team was booked into a Cincinnati tournament and yours was running at the Kentucky Horse Park in Lexington, your Mom shuttled between the two.

"High Investment" Parents

You were lucky to have parents who had their eye on your future. They figured out who you were and what your gifts were. They found ways of working with your best motivations — mostly by doing things with you when you were little. That is how you learned to love to work: Doing it with Mom or Dad was fun! So today you are loving your school work and your contact sports, and you manage to volunteer at the emergency room. Work is fun! That means that your whole adult career is going to feel like a game. You will sometimes want to apologize to your employer for paying you — you enjoy everything you do as much as if it were recreation.

When you were only six years old, your daddy recruited you to help with spring housecleaning on a beautiful Saturday. Every room got sorted, organized, and cleaned. And your dad showed you how to do the vacuum cleaning with the magic wand as you dragged the cannister from room to room.

The next morning, Sunday, barely daylight, your Dad awakened to the sounds of vacuum cleaning. He and your mom were startled to find you up, dressed and touching up the living area where you spotted some disorder. No wonder you are an empowered young woman who loves to keep yourself and everything around you "just right." You learned it early and learned it well.

Girls who are "latch key" kids and daughters in single parent families are either vulnerable to trouble or catch the opportunity to pull a lot of the household load early. With a little coaching, these women whip out household work, keep the place picked up and orderly and come into responsibility ahead of their time. When parents praise them and thank God for them, the motivation often carries them through in grand shape.

High Value Daughter

From the first, you knew your parents were going to teach you everything they knew. They had no secrets when you had questions. Somewhere about age ten, you knew that you were getting big chunks of responsibility. You could do almost anything that had to be done around the house. Your parents had worked with you so that you could have survived, even then, if they had been flat in bed suddenly sick. Everything out of doors was familiar to you. Only driving the car was off limits. But with your careful training on lawn equipment, even that was only inches away from your skills.

A pair of beautiful twin girls near us got the surprise of their lives on their sixteenth birthday: monogrammed key rings containing house and car keys. They don't even have drivers' licenses, but their Dad said, "We want you to know that being sixteen is special, and that we trust you. So carry the keys to remind you that we are in this whole thing together and we celebrate your growing up."

You answered the phone knowing exactly what to tell people who were trying to reach one of your parents. Sometimes, when the caller stated the problem, you knew what your dad or mom would say, and you offered the information.

When you goofed, nobody panicked. Whichever parent was on hand would simply keep you focused on your own future, and say, "What do you wish you had done instead?"

You exploded a few times, angry at your parents but mostly at the feeling that your own independent future was so far away. Even then, your parents wouldn't fight with you. They could have, because you were temporarily pretty rotten to them. But they had their eye on your future and knew that dealing with anger is a lifelong responsibility. So they offered you options, asked questions, and finally said, "You choose. Take your time. Whatever you are feeling is OK, but it is not OK to treat people like garbage. So cool down, then tell us what decision you have made among the options we've all brainstormed."

I've been describing here the "Intimate Family" which places a high value on everybody in the house. And in that family every member has more and more responsibilities. Everyone knows they are free to choose. Those choices will affect other members of the family, so they have to be good choices — choices with consequences that are easy to live with.

Some girls grow up in "Competing Families" in which there is always tension over who decides, who gets the best stuff and who controls everybody else.

Others live in "Chaotic Families" where nobody seems to care whether anybody has basic needs met or has a future of any kind — every kid and parent for themselves!

Even more girls live in "Showcase Families" where the emphasis is on "looking good" to outsiders, and that can cause a lot of stress. In these families, one person makes almost all decisions and also decides what to "showcase." That can keep everyone pretty tense, and lead to dishonesty with true feelings. It's common for kids to feel "used" in order to make the family "look good."

Intimate families, in contrast, are not embarrassed about anybody in the family. Everybody is valued, and the family's reputation is really in everybody's hands. This means that the risk of living with the consequences of their choices is a risk everybody knows is worth taking. There is a high investment in teaching the children everything they need to know, and everything about the parent's beliefs, values and decisions. So nobody worries about occasional poor decisions, because they can be remedied some way.

Fantastic Dad

Girls desperately need their fathers at a couple of points in their journey from conception to living on their own. From birth to about six years old, girls mimic their femininity as they imitate their mothers. But from the beginning, and especially when they are hitting middle school years, they "rehearse" their femininity and womanly behaviors in dealing with their fathers.

Fathers polish their daughters' femininity, or sex role, by serving as rehearsal directors, from about age 10 until their daughters are launched as responsible, gracious and good women. During these teen and early adult years, a young woman often feels that her daddy understands her, affirms her, believes in her in ways that her mother does not. During these years mothers often feel left out as the girl charges her batteries for transformation into an adult woman. These are "rehearsal symptoms" in healthy families.

Healthy fathers are available to daughters, but would die rather than see them violated or become abusive themselves. Check out Chapter 8 for ways of dealing with damaged trust in worst case situations.

Here, again, if a girl misses her father, or if Dad is too busy, gone too much, is an abuser or an alcoholic or is otherwise caught up in his own problems or his career, the young girl and woman can suffer seriously. Girls are most damaged if the father absence occurred before birth or very early, but the symptoms rarely show until she hits pubescence. So it is easy to believe that having a daddy you can trust is especially important when you embrace your adult womanhood.

Girls who make up their minds to learn everything they can about the adult world of a responsible male will automatically pick model surrogate fathers outside the home. They hang around with a friend whose dad makes a priority of being a father who is affirming and available to his daughter. Or they get involved in soccer, church clubs, symphony or summer athletics and check out a safe and continuing substitute father off whom they can bounce their femininity. Since very few men teach in kindergarten or elementary school, it is sometimes hard for girls to find good men outside volunteer programs at church, summer recreation or community clubs.

Girls whose healthy, available fathers contribute to a stable, consistent childhood with discipline, affirmation and a feeling of safety tend to be able to do these things:

1. They can make moral judgments based on everybody having special value, and on keeping relationships honest.

Chapter Three: Check Those Roots!

2. They find it easy to believe in God — in the unity and order of the universe.
3. They can adopt rigorous self-discipline to achieve goals they choose — even if it means saving, waiting or going against the flow of the popularity scene.
4. They are able to make commitments to people and to affirm membership in communities of faith and service.
5. Evaluating a potential husband and making a commitment to life-long exclusive love and marriage will come easily.

The single best predictor for a woman's healthy adult life is the quality of her relationship with her father. She will be confident in her own self directly in proportion to how her father valued her and respected her. She will be able to evaluate quality and safety in a man directly in relationship to how much integrity and positive treatment her Dad gave her. Her ability to tackle work, mothering and a meaningful sense of vocation as a woman is profoundly related to how her father affirmed her during her childhood and teen years. No wonder you are lucky to have had a fantastic Dad!

Maximum Mother

You were really a lucky girl. You knew long before I could describe it that your parents and your family are your "First Curriculum" for growing up healthy and secure as an adult.

A girl needs about a dozen years of consistent mothering by a good woman who provides warmth, discipline, praise and a lot of visible demonstration of what a woman is and how she lives and moves in the world. If her mother doesn't meet these needs, she is often hurt or at least underdeveloped in some predictable ways. But with a healthy relationship and plenty of mother availability, you will find that you automatically have these gifts:

1. You easily trust other people in basic friendships and social contact.
2. You can express complicated feelings, and are ready to join and make commitments to community, church and marriage.
3. You will feel confident in your developing womanhood which has blossomed as you imitated her ways, learning how to walk, work, talk and relate to other people in sex-appropriate ways.

4. You will have learned how to make good judgments about men and will know how to relate to a man positively.

You have been lucky, for sure. Many girls get a lot more criticism than affirmation from their parents. When Mom isn't able to give good discipline and feedback to a girl, childhood can be torture. An alcoholic or otherwise abusing mother creates a vacuum in which a girl simply does not get the "first curriculum" of how to be a woman. If she feels cheated by her mother, she is especially vulnerable to becoming an angry young woman and may repeat her mother's behavior which she has learned at home. Losing your mother to alcohol or any other compulsive pattern when you hit your teens can send a young woman to search out a substitute mom. You will need mother affirmation before pubescence, and need it badly, but for the rest of your life your "Mom connection" is easily the most important for stabilizing your sense of being loved and of being secure and safe.

It would be easy to imagine that either a mother or a father could get you ready for all of life. And single parents certainly get my high praise when they must carry the whole parenting load alone. But the fact is that most parenting is done spontaneously and unconsciously. Mothers simply do their parenting work without thinking about what they are doing as they show you how to be a woman. And fathers usually do their work spontaneously, too. If either of them must "be a parent for the other parent" or "do the whole parenting job alone," they tend to face a lot of work. So you were lucky, indeed, to have both parents doing their spontaneous parenting with you. To show you how "easily" they do their work, let me tell you some things that happened to you very early.

Dads and Moms Together

If anybody had seen your actual birth, they would have seen you held tightly in your mother's arms very soon. Mothers encompass their babies the same way everywhere in the world. Fathers simply cannot hold a baby in that same way for very long, but mothers do it instinctively. Mothers do that encircling embrace in a way that looks like magic. Mothers keep doing this encompassing at almost every contact with a child until the child is old enough to wiggle out of her grasp and get loose on the floor. Mothers tend to want to cuddle you to fix anything that goes wrong. As long as you are a mother's child, even if she lives until you are eighty-five, she will encompass you if she can.

There is a famous marble sculpture done by Michelangelo called *The Pieta*. It shows Mary holding the dead body of the adult Jesus as he is taken down from the cross. Michelangelo sculpted Mary in the cuddling, rocking position, holding her adult Son as if he were still her baby. Mothers rarely hold you like that after you are ten or twelve years old, but their encompassing love still surrounds you in much the same way their arms once did. Robert Munsch has captured this encompassing mother image in the amazing children's book titled *Love You Forever.*

What your dad did for you was a very different thing. Dads hold the baby out in front of them to look in the little newborn's eyes. As the baby gets more strength, fathers hold their babies at arms' length, move them up and down and around, always face to face, and do these wonderful games with them. This is called engrossing behavior. You can see why dads are more likely to finally say, "My daughter is ready to go away to college," or "Our gal can make it on her own. Look at the good decisions she has been making since she was ten." Dads have been rehearsing this separateness, this autonomy, from their child's birth. Dads' ease of separation has been shown as early as the day of birth simply by the way they hold their babies.

In an equally opposite way, your mom helped you to develop relationships, to attach, to value other people. But your dad is more committed to integrity, honesty, justice and fairness. He can sniff out deception or dishonesty in people and protect you from their exploitation. The best moral development research shows these differing centers of value: relationships for women and justice for men. So you need healthy doses of both father and mother experiences.

Brothers

Girls are lucky to have brothers. It doesn't always seem lucky, but it is, actually. Girls who have brothers as well as a father know better how to deal with men. And if you are in a healthy family, you know that girls are as important as boys, and that they deserve freedom, responsibility and trust just as boys do. If you had an older brother, you likely got an extra dose of fathering from him.

OK, because if you had younger brothers and sisters, you likely did your part in mothering them. We all do it — almost from birth.

It is not uncommon for a sister-brother relationship to feel a little like parent-to-child or child-to-parent. But brothers, whether older or younger, are "other." So you will remember times when there was a tremendous advantage to having a brother, and at other times he was like an outsider, an intruder.

Men and boys think and work in ways that baffle women and girls. So you will have had good practice in dealing with "the male perspective" if you were able to handle the brother-sister relationship without either of you going crazy. Brothers are different from fathers. Fathers know they are responsible for you and they build bridges of understanding to you. Brothers rarely take the time to be so kind to you.

Sisters

You were only 14 months old when your sister was born. She was almost your first doll — a real one. My early Nikon shots of the two of you outfitted almost alike are stunning. What a lovely pair of granddaughters!

But you needed space. She was, as us older folk say, "colicky" for six months. And I'm afraid we all turned most of our attention to her in her daily discomfort. But when we discovered you again — this serious, care-tender older sister, we saw you were wonderfully introverted and able to help with the mothering in an amazing way.

The sister, however, was a free spirit. She got the attention for both of you for a few months, and it saw her through some painful early months. Today she is brightly extraverted — living in her outer world, thriving on friendships and social activity.

But the two of you are now women together. You understand each other in a way that would make it easy to conspire on any deal. Soccer stars together, going separate ways with ballet and piano, you come together again as you chart your high school careers. And when there is conflict — I imagine, but have never seen it — you may mount a stiffer battle because you are both wired as women. Your sense of violated rights, space and feelings — especially when relationships or privacy are violated — set off a very visibly different dynamic than we see between brothers or between a brother and a sister. There is "no vengeance like a woman's" is simply a warning that women care more and therefore are capable of more global shaking wrath than we typically see in men.

In families where each child is valued the same and where everybody is learning all of the secrets of managing the house, the meals and the whole show inside and out, sisters can be very different. One can be an athlete and the other a musician, and everybody can be healthy and know everybody else is supportive. In the showcase, chaotic or competing household, however, ugly things can go on between children and often it is one of the girls who becomes the family scapegoat. If that happens, she is the victim who catches ridicule, shame and sarcasm. This kind of family life tells us the whole family is sick, and needs help. Bible stories of Cain and Abel and Jacob and Esau remind us of tragic things that happen between brothers in conflict. Usually such families today need outside help — a pastor, a doctor or a counselor — to get their eyes on the really important things: everybody's exquisite value and the importance of keeping present problems focused on solutions that buy the future and guarantee a healthy adult life for every child.

Adopted kids mixed with natural kids, or a blended family of any sort, seem to predict that somebody will feel like a scapegoat victim more often than in traditional families.

Family

Dad and Mom, of course, are models and referees at the same time. So the health in your family tells us that they have shown all of you how to be responsible men and women, and that you are all good learners. But they have provided ground rules to protect everybody in the same way. Their "no sarcasm, no violence, talk it out and tell your feelings" strategies have given you a lot of strength as a new woman.

All families have conflicts and tears, and every member of a family will sometime be violated by other people in the family. But you have been lucky to be under the roof of a family that has kept its pain up to date and has not allowed anyone to suffer day after day. This has been a wonderful gift from your family. And you are wearing it beautifully. The two words to describe that gift are "security" and "responsibility." The next chapter is a celebration of those gifts.

Chapter Four

Dreams Do Come True!

There was the Christmas, now so long ago, when we negotiated with your families for permission to outfit each of you with your very own Cabbage Patch doll. We checked eyes and hair color. After all, the dolls came with a birth certificate, so they needed to be your very own babies.

And you gave us such special moments! There was the evening when the three of you little girls — about four through six — lined up to get the Rose Milk lotion squeezed into your little hands. You and Grandma rubbed it gently into your hands and faces at bedtime. When Grandma offered Rose Milk to Jason, older than all of you, he blurted out his masculine rejection: "No way!" and bolted from the room.

Now there are adult career and love imaginations dancing in your heads. The seasons of life bring new agendas. So I'm urging you to dream the very best.

Here's Your Dream License!

I want to give you permission to reflect, to imagine yourself being the person you most want to become and doing the things you most admire in an adult woman. Here are some questions to put you in touch with your imagination. Give yourself permission to be aware of your deepest longings and dreams.

1. Add 10 years to your age now. Imagine that you are on stage before a large crowd of people. What are you doing, with the

whole world watching? When the hazy fog of your teen years lifts, what is the life-long image you have of yourself?
2. Who are the people you see on stage with you in your 10-year vision? How did they get into your imagination? What is their relationship to you in the picture you see?

Young Women Who Speak Out

It has always been true: Healthy young folks always have their eye on the future. On the day the Christian movement was launched, look at the words in the inauguration speech delivered by Peter (who was quoting the prophet Joel) as recorded in Acts 2:14-21, and ask yourself whether you are becoming the kind of outspoken healthy woman who can celebrate good and confront evil whenever someone needs to speak out prophetically:

> "In the last days, God says,
> I will pour out my Spirit on all people.
> Your sons and daughters will prophesy,
> your young men will see visions,
> your old men will dream dreams.
> Even on my servants both men and women,
> I will pour out my Spirit in those days,
> and they will prophesy."

There is one vision, especially, that young women consistently see. This is true of religious women, but it is also true of those who may not be aware of a hunger for faith in God. The same vision shows up in children from poverty and from wealth. Even girls who have been abused or abandoned almost always have the same dream: *Somewhere there is a good man with whom I can share all of my secrets for the rest of my life.* I call this the "exclusive, life-long intimacy dream." You may find yourself even praying a desperate prayer that somewhere God is keeping some young man free from the crazy things that are everywhere going wrong in the world — saving him for you sometime in the future. Your Grandma and I pray that prayer for you all the time.

Hang On to Your Self!

Carol Gilligan at Harvard is studying girls' development. She finds that at about age 12, most girls "abandon themselves." She talks with sixth grade girls and their teachers and finds that something happens that causes girls to stop being confident about themselves. They tend to give up during classroom debate, and to distrust their own judgment. This happens in school, especially. And it happens to girls with women teachers as well as when men are the teachers. It seems to be something that girls do to themselves as much as it is something that we do to them. Let me describe some of the things young girls seem to be abandoning:

1. *They give up their curiosity and love of learning.* Evidently they decide that doing well in school is a handicap. Smart girls are not respected by other girls, and they are a threat to boys who want to compete for top spots academically.

2. *They give up their vision of vocation, career, high achievement and special training.* Girls tend to take their maturing sexual development as a signal to look for Mr. Wonderful, become a wife and mother and leave the dreaming to him. Fatherhood can boost a young man's career, but motherhood seems to end a young woman's life dream, unless her husband conspires with her to keep it alive.

3. *They forfeit their sense of gifts and vocation beyond marriage and motherhood.* A sensitive husband will try to keep his young wife's dream alive: "What training do you want to get? What energizes you? After the babies are up and out of the nest, what will you want to be about?"

So get your long-range vision set. Anchor it in your high school and college interests. Get preliminary credentials on line. Swap dreams with your young "Mr. Wonderful," partly to see whether he really values you as a person, and to let him see that you are not going to roll over and die if he abandons you now or ever. Marriage based on dependency is always deformed. When "two become one," it is urgent that they be whole numbers both before and after they come together. When "two become one" nobody gets cancelled out. Across a lifetime there will be times when either of you may have to take a lion's share of responsibility in the event of death or disability of the partner.

In the beautiful doctrine of Creation, God gave authority and dominion to "them." The man and the woman were given complete responsibility for decisions and management of this planet. We read it wrong when we get the idea that the man is to dominate the woman. "He shall rule over her" is the awful report of the effects of failure in Eden. Any male who controls, overrules or otherwise dominates a woman is living out the original sin. And any woman who gives up while adoring her man is equally guilty of loving too much — the woman's original sin.

Take Your Feelings Seriously!

I have known for all of my adult life that healthy and religious girls grow up with a dream of exclusive, life-long intimacy with one man forever. But Robert Coles and Geoffrey Stokes, reporting on their research with teens from 1,025 *Rolling Stone Magazine* subscriber homes, found the same dream driving even the non-religious teens. Their book is *Sex and the American Teenager.*

Those secular researchers were baffled to find that young love expects the first love will be the *only* love of a lifetime. I am not surprised. It was true with me at 15 and when I lost that first love, I didn't reach out again until I found Robbie when I was 18; we were married just before I was 20. Healthy folks are able to make profoundly deep life-long commitments and to make them early. "Casual dating" or "dating around" is evidently not what healthy young men and women want. Both are created for commitment and intimacy, and the loss or failure of a developing relationship is a serious and painful experience. They know instinctively to shut down and go into intentional grieving when they lose an important friendship they had hoped would develop into life-long marriage. "Blessed are those who grieve, for they will be healed of their loss" is an important footnote for you, if you want to rebuild your dream after a loss.

Going for Your Dream

If you have a pretty clear vision of who you are becoming and what kind of person your ideal man will be, then you will take time to build the dream deliberately and well. Here are some things that have always been true about building an exclusive, life-long intimate relationship.

1. *Intimacy is a harvest of patient months and years of getting acquainted.* Get to know the person well. If you want a life-long marriage, check him out as a person to see who he really is. Meet his parents and grandparents. Find out where he came

Chapter Four: Dreams Do Come True! 41

from on his family tree, and whether he is healthy, happy and decent with everybody. True intimacy always grows slowly out of the solid soil of knowing each other casually and intently. All of the great Bible stories about loving couples speaks about "knowing" as better then mere loving.

This means dozens, perhaps hundreds, of hours watching and listening as the admired person moves within the same group you do. Marriages fail at alarming rates when the partners try to become physically intimate without "knowing" each other well before the sexual fires are ignited. They may quickly kiss and touch or even be sexual, but they will be creating a bubble, not a solid real intimate relationship.

2. *Intentionally keep your developing relationship in public to guarantee that knowledge accumulates well ahead of intimacy.*

Intimacy is the goal, the pay off, and it is the cement of a powerful "life-long, exclusive marriage." But premature intimacy or *pseudo intimacy* almost always explodes, leaving two victims with wounds that often haunt their marriages later. So, if you are living in pursuit of that vision of yours, be sure that you are getting to know the person without complicating the relationship with premature intimacy.

3. *Keep your relationship in public and under family visibility to keep your "real world time" in sync with your "intimacy world time."*

From about age 15 on, your intimacy hunger may be ready to eat the calendar and grab the man of your dreams. And with the energy and time you can muster, you could develop a fully ripened relationship and be ready for consummation in a year or two. What this tells you is that biologically you are healthy and that you have a high priority for intimacy.

But the real world calendar of schooling, family resources and emotional maturity may be running somewhere behind your biological and intimacy calendar. Be candid with your parents if your two calendars are badly out of sync. They may be able to endorse an earlier "real world" calendar than you imagined. But for most of us, the only way to synchronize those two calendars is to contract with each other and with our families to guarantee that the relationship has no absolute privacy. Count on it; no one is immune from this rule: Absolute privacy predicts premature intimacy!

4. *Your competency as a mature person is being built as you take responsibility for the relationship and the welfare and value of the other person; this is your most important life curriculum.*

The pleasures of intimacy are so good and so compelling that they provide the test of your responsibility as no other life experience can. The responsibility test covers such things as these:
- Your honesty.
- Your ability to postpone premature intimacy.
- Your willingness to take full emotional responsibility for your partner.
- Your readiness to take full legal and public responsibility for your relationship.

You will not be surprised to read everywhere that the divorce rate of couples who lived together and later marry runs more than double the divorce rate of those who keep full responsibility and full intimacy locked together in a public marriage. It could be that something was lost by the premature sexual intimacy. But it is more likely that there is a deep character flaw and that this lack of trust eats like leprosy in their relationship. Those couples who lived together before marriage did not take full public and legal responsibility for each other, so they evidently fear that their partner, who exploited them without public ceremony or serious contract, will abandon them now or later.

Beyond this lack of trust, there is another serious problem with premature sexual experience. Everyone develops an appetite for sexual intimacy, and it is powerfully shaped by first love sexual experience.

If your first love sexual experience is wrapped in the excitement of unmarried, secret or forbidden pleasure you will experience both sexual pleasure and an adrenaline high because of this set of risks you have deliberately taken. Sex in marriage is likely, then, to seem flat and unexciting. So you will be very vulnerable to having an affair which can produce the same adrenaline high you experienced in your first premature, high-risk sexual adventure. Premarriage sex very often leads to dull sex after the wedding. And this adrenaline high is the obvious reason. Your sexual appetite thinks the high

Chapter Four: Dreams Do Come True!

feeling is part of sexual intimacy even though the high really works against intimacy and encourages addiction to high-risk sex.

Couples who synchronize their responsibility and their intimacy forge a bond in the crucible of real world experience. Intimacy carries its own high without risk-produced adrenaline. Those who discover intimacy find that they are excellent lovers not only when they are on vacation, but day by day. They enjoy being sexual without props or fantasy episodes, even in the middle of meeting payments, working long hours, sitting up with sick children and facing the whole agenda of real life.

So go for your dream! Check him out, of course. Really get to know him — first at a distance, then in the traffic as you watch him operate in casual group environments. Don't imagine that if he orders you around, dominates you and embarrasses you now he will treat you any better after the wedding.

Getting to know him slowly will let you set him free if he does not share your commitment to mutual respect, consensus decisions and building on each other's strengths. If both of you respect each other and live honestly before your families, count on it: You will be able to handle the responsibility of a slowly ripening intimacy.

Chapter Five

Getting to Know Each Other—in Public, Slowly

In the CBS-Fox version of *Les Miserables*, a powerful picture of young-love bonding occurs as Cosette is spotted by Marius, a young man of 16 or so who is caught up in the French Revolution. You can see it in his eyes as he first catches sight of her in a park at a political rally. He pursues her by secretly getting a note to her at her mansion by wrapping it around a rock thrown over the gate.

In this John Gay adaptation of the Victor Hugo classic, Cosette's response is equally magnetic. She and her father, who is brought into the plot, attempt to escape from Paris to England and to take the young boy with them. But he is unable to borrow money from his grandfather to make the trip. The old man gives him enough money to buy a new hat — suggesting that he groom himself appropriate to his aristocratic ancestry. When the wealthy old nobleman discovers that Marius is in love, he mocks him: "Why marry her? Make her your mistress, instead!"

With that insult to his integrity, Marius throws the money at his grandfather's feet, whirls and runs away. And it is Cosette's father who, failing to make the escape to England, joins the battle that emerges, rescues wounded young Marius and nurses him back to life — for Cosette and himself and the heroic quality of pure young love. Finally, the movie ends with the small but grace-filled wedding of two young folks in love.

Catch the old 1978 classic movie, if you can. Today's video and Hollywood love stories tend to be of wounded and warped people who establish quick and steamy sexual liaisons and who live faithless lives across many relationships, never finding peace and fidelity in love. If those broken images of love have caught up with you, be sure to turn to Chapter 8, "Coming Back When Things Go Wrong," and re-capture your vision of hope and innocence again.

The Mystery of Bonding

When I mention bonding, I'm not talking about a special glue you buy at the craft shop or even of what your dentist may do in repairing a broken tooth. By bonding I refer to the powerful attachment which occurs between people when they have long-term or powerful experiences together. The high emotion we feel at special times evidently triggers chemicals in the brain which highlight or emotionally mark some experience unlike any other we have had.

Parent-child attachment is easy to understand because of the time they invest in close contact. And birth bonding enhances the parent-child relationship for a lifetime. We now know that the first two and a half hours of life are critical bonding minutes for both parents and the newborn baby. One result of good birth bonding is that both the parents and the baby are more peaceable with each other. The baby cries less, and the parents worry about the child less if they have skin, eye and voice contact in spontaneous exchange during that critical first couple of hours. The brain chemicals released in the emotional high of those first minutes of life do the bonding. We are attached in these peak bonding experiences to the people who will always be special to us.

Friends are often bonded by painful experiences. Victims of a hurricane or an earthquake or hostages taken prisoner often develop amazingly strong attachments which bring them together in annual reunions for the rest of their lives.

But "pair bonding" is the best of bonding. This bonding looks very much like birth bonding. In fact, young adults are likely to make pair bonds that closely resemble the strength of the bonding they had with their parents as young children. A well-bonded adult from a healthy family, for example, breaks away from childhood dependency, becomes free and forms a marriage bond easily. These healthy teens or young adults rarely get involved in ugly power struggles with their parents.

Father Absence and Bonding

You can almost always predict what kind of a marriage partner anyone is going to make by listening to the way they talk with, talk about and deal with their parents. If a young man is consistently in high voltage emotional tension with his mother, you can count on this: If you marry him, he will treat you no better than he treats his mother. This is true of boys who have been emotionally abused as well as of those who simply never quite found a way to win their mother's affirmation in healthy ways. Boys depend, too, on early and life-long affirmation from their fathers. So a young man who has lost a parent or is in high conflict with parents may be emotionally unable to treat you with respect. You may find you are doing a lot of parenting in your relationship, or taking a lot of orders and other emotional abuse. These are pretty good signs that the young man is hurting and needs more help than you can provide in a friendship or a marriage.

You may find yourself uncertain. On the one hand, the guy treats you well, is eager to be close, to touch and be touched. And when two young people get together, both of whom are wounded by emotional abuse or abandonment, they easily mix parenting comfort with affection, and the result is usually a very mixed up friendship.

On the other hand, a healthy young man is putting some peaceful distance between his parents and himself. Somewhere deep in his soul he longs for love and an exclusive life-long relationship. In this appropriately starved state, he is likely to welcome the easily available woman with her need to be cuddled, kissed and touched. If the young woman is wounded by father neglect or absence, she may prematurely trigger intimate physical contact. A healthy young couple, however, if they are not physically turned on by inappropriate or seductive intimacy, tend to move slowly and exclusively in their pursuit of marriage.

The really troubled boys have begun long ago to "macho" themselves. They decided not to risk being hurt again, so they move through gestures that look like love, but actually reveal their hollow and hurting souls in ways you can detect. Here are some of their symptoms:

1. Macho males speak the language of love, but they brag to their friends about how they are exploiting you.

2. They control a woman. This may look like care giving, but if it includes dominance, control and impatience, you will know he is a wounded macho male.
3. A macho man will keep up a good show in public, but may seem to be somebody not quite so nice in private.
4. The macho is out for what he can get and protects himself from considering your needs, your identity and your interests.
5. If your macho male has been abused, he will likely splash shame on you, blaming you for anything that goes wrong.
6. He will run the whole show; his final words will be "Don't call me. I'll call you." He is preoccupied with never being dumped, but he casually dumps his women.

A macho man needs help, and he almost never can accept it from the close friend in a dating relationship. Don't imagine that you can fix him by living up to his demands. You will become a codependent, dancing the dance of his warped needs and taking the blame for his emptiness and pain.

Crazy Bonding

Crazy bonding happens in families or couples when they mix any form of abuse, stress or control into the relationship. If any person is so needy as to manipulate, to control by jealousy or rage or to control the relationship consistently to meet his or her own needs, the bonding is flawed. If there is abuse — emotional, physical or sexual — the bond is often cemented with super glue! I call it crazy bonding because even though the relationship is destructive, neither person seems able to get out of it.

Abused or crazy-bonded children, for example, often cannot leave home to go to college or live far away from their abusing parents as adults. They are always coming home to the abuse, choosing the abuse they know back home instead of risking the wild world of imagined abuse they do not know. Abused children tend to be more dependent, and eventually are more likely to be carbon copies of the abuser. They are almost sure to be abusers when it is their turn. So avoid the dance of crazy bonding.

If you are a daughter of divorce or have survived in an alcohol abusing household, or if you have been shaken by any other emotionally devastating experience, you may want to look at Chapter

Chapter Five: Getting to Know Each Other

Eight. It is entitled "Coming Back When Things Go Wrong." Then, come back, because I'm going to share the secrets I know about how to develop a life-long, exclusive bond with that man of your best visions!

Healthy Bonding

I want to outline the best of all possible pair bonding scenarios for you. These steps or progressive phases of bonding intimacy will unfold slowly and completely for you. You do not need to study them in a book or to memorize the sequence. Simply be an honest and healthy woman, take your time and watch the mystery of the pair bond unfold.

I've adapted Desmond Morris' "twelve steps" of pair bonding for you. He presents them in his book *Intimate Behavior*. I describe them in this chapter and the next, dividing the 12 steps into two major parts.

Your life-long exclusive marriage will find you enjoying *all of the twelve steps* for the rest of your life. They arrive one-at-a-time, slowly and progressively. But once you have completed your work on a single step, it potentially belongs to the two of you forever — unless the entire structure collapses and you are devastated with the losses involved.

There are actually four levels of bonding, with three steps each. They include these unfolding opportunities:

Steps 1 Through 6

A. The entry gate to a potential life-long relationship.
B. Building the foundations for exclusive commitment.

Steps 7 Through 12

C. The interior mansion your bonded marriage will inhabit and furnish for a lifetime.
D. The exclusive citadel and private chamber appears last and is absolutely protected, safe and exclusive.

Notice that the first six steps need to be built in public. They *require* public surveillance not only to keep you going slowly on the road to ultimate intimacy, but to remind you of the wonderful choice the two of you are making — when compared with the rest of the folks around. This public environment for the life-long bond, where people can see you day after day as you display that you have chosen each other in the crowd is crucial for the life-long bond.

We will look at those first two sets of three steps here.

Entry Gate to the Pair Bond

Remember that these bonding steps are not something somebody invented to teach you how to make an exclusive, life-long bond. These steps are what careful observers have found are true everywhere, in every culture, when a woman and a man form that mysterious, life-long exclusive bond. So, if you have felt the first rush of attraction for a special person you will recognize the powerful and good sequence of the "Entry Gate" as you look at the first three steps:

1. *Eye to body.* "Wow! Where have I been? Has he stepped out of heaven just for me?" There's a sudden rush of surprise and excitement. He may have grown up next door or have moved in from Orlando. It makes little difference. He will look new and special. When Cupid strikes with the arrow of *eros*, it is pure adoration, and it captures your full attention. There may have been flocks of prospects before. Now he is your singular vision. Nobody on earth compares with him at this moment.

Unless you have been sexually abused or are the victim of our pornographic culture, there will be no sexual content to this first sighting. There will be plenty of sexual imagination later, but not now. You sense that you do not yet *know* him, and that task of getting to know him is what pulls your eyes out of their sockets trying to fill up your senses with this vision of possibilities for the rest of your life.

2. *Eye to eye.* In the crowded place someone else is looking. He is enveloping you with his eyes. *What good timing,* you think! And helping to make it happen is the fact that through the mystery of the small brain voltage which passes through the eyes, you can almost always turn someone's eyes to you — simply by looking at them. "I feel like somebody is watching me" is often more than a feeling, it's a reality. So you turn instinctively to meet a pair of eyes!

I'll walk you later through the great love passages of the Bible, but sneak a preview now if you like by looking at the ways Song of Songs reports this adoration of the eyes: In the New International

Version, 1:16 says, "How handsome you are, my lover! Oh, how charming!" Or look at 2:3-4, "Like an apple tree among the trees of the forest is my lover among the young men. I delight to sit in his shade, and his fruit is sweet to my taste. He has taken me to the banquet hall, and his banner over me is love."

3. *Voice to voice.* When the eyes have met, all civilizations require a next step. However clumsily you do it, you must speak to him. First you may want to locate someone who knows both of you. "What is his name?" you long to know. If you are very lucky there is a gracious gift of an introduction offered by the mutual acquaintance. But you will find a way. Your honest eyes will find him involuntarily, and he will read them infallibly. Words will come honestly, too — gentle words of casual friendship and common interest. Friends always create space into which the other can come and find respect and acceptance.

Eventually you will look over the families. You will know you are in a serious friendship when you are eager for your parents and family members to meet him. As grandparents, Robbie and I are wonderfully affirmed when you say, "Can you come to my soccer game Saturday. There is somebody I want you to meet and he is going to be there."

Life-long relationships need a slow start. Remember that building a healthy friendship is always enhanced if you can develop it in the presence of trusted friendships. You won't be surprised to know that in Spanish culture the engagement must follow this intense eye contact. It is a crime in that Moorish culture to look intently at a person to whom you are not engaged or married!

You can take it from there. Count on it: If he was gazing at you, he will be able to respond if you find your voice first. Both of you will feel healthier, more complete, as you take charge with quiet dignity. In the worst case scenario young girls are likely to pull a prank, drop a bag of popcorn or create a scene in which the first speech is out of embarrassment or retaliation. Perhaps any speaking is better than none, but immature social moves rarely get anybody off toward a significant search for the life-long exclusive relationship we all long for.

The voice-to-voice phase sets in motion the communication so critical in the healthy development of a bonded marriage. Men who have not established a reputation for being verbal suddenly find they can talk. I've known boys who had hardly composed one complete sentence in a year around their parents who suddenly burst into coherent speech with a girl. Silent types are no longer silent. You'll know that bonding is working when suddenly the two of you find words to speak. What is more, both of you may be evoked to write love notes, even poetry. Do it! Develop your communication and affectional skills while the motivation is bubbling up and overflowing. They will serve you very well for the remainder of a rich lifetime.

And use the telephone. Talking is more important than being under the stress of dating. Write notes, letters, friendship messages, poetry and songs. Give yourself permission to put your attention into language.

Foundations for the Pair Bond

The next three steps involve simple and light touching. Desmond Morris and Melvin Konner, both of whom have studied pair bonding in many animal and bird species as well as among humans, are able to describe how important the bonding ritual is. Konner, in *The Tangled Wing: Biological Constraints on the Human Spirit*, for example, observes that among the "exclusively monogamous pair bonding species," the pair bonding ritual is very deliberate, with plenty of opportunity for either one to abandon the relationship. In exclusive monogamous bird species the courtship ritual includes building the nest. Everything is completed before breeding occurs.

I sometimes think maybe God created all species exclusively monogamous — one male with one female. But it seems evil damaged most of the species and their ability to bond exclusively. With human marriages breaking up in tragic numbers, we may decide it is worthwhile to pay attention to our inner vision and deep longings for exclusive, life-long marriage. If we do that, we will meet our own needs and will build the bond slowly, deliberately and with profound respect for the non-renewable resource of ourselves.

You must guard against following some clever scheme into becoming prematurely sexual. Anybody can come up with a secret plan to get sexual experience. Only intentional people come up with plans to postpone it until it is guaranteed exclusive and life long. As the relationship matures, you will still find pleasure in visually sighting each other, in eye-to-eye contact and in endless voice-to-voice talking. Look at these foundation steps in the pair bonding sequence.

4. *Hand-to-hand.* First touch between a man and a woman is almost always the touch of hands. In a crowd, the hands touch in order not to lose each other. Reaching out for each other is automatic: The hands link up. Even though the reaching out is for the practical reason of hanging on — to cross the street, to negotiate the traffic as you rush toward seating at the concert or to be sure of places together in the choir or the auditorium — the electric sensation that strikes you when hands touch is a bonding touch.

There is this magic with every new step in the bonding sequence, but first touch is sure to trigger its chemical high. The brain releases endorphins which instantly set off tingling sensations centered in your chest. These breath-taking stirrings are often felt near the sternum in the middle of your chest. It's common for the sensations to make you catch your breath suddenly as if you need more air. The brain chemicals are bonding the moment in permanent memory. If we could combine this kind of brain chemistry with academic studies, we could remember everything!

The hands will always be important in your relationship, so it is right that they are the first connection. By some estimates, one-third of all of your nerve endings are wired through in your hands. Human hands are especially created for communication. Beware the person who uses hands of affection to slap, punch or beat you!

5. *Arm-to-shoulder.* Desmond Morris found that all humans next take steps to connect in a first ownership gesture by which one of the pair will pull the other close to the side. This pull to a lock-step side-by-side posture occurs by vice gripping the arm around the partner's shoulder. Notice that both are still facing forward, as in hand-to-hand, but the gesture tells everyone that this is a couple! High and visible, the arm around the shoulder is a body link that serves notice on everyone present that these are joining in a special way. If they are of approximate equal height, the arms often entwine as both of the partners vice-lock the other's shoulders. As with the hands, this posture brings with it enormous brain chemical enjoyment. "I am loved, I am wanted, I have value!" is always an occasion for celebration.

6. *Arm-to-waist.* Now the vice-lock releases, the hand limply falls to the waist. When both partners take this posture, the elbows cross behind their backs and the couple is "X-linked" together. It is common now for their heads to tuck down. They seem to be studying the ground a lot. They pull away from the crowd. They seem oblivious to other people. At Step 3, voice-to-voice, they were on the phone to each other, sometimes endlessly. Now they are talking, talking, talking — while locked in the Step 6 X-link.

While the Step 3 voice contact focused endlessly on gossipy nothing things their parents would have thought trivial, the conversation now is dead serious. It is serious because it is clearing the way for "till death do us part" kinds of plans and promises. The conversation has a perpetual "what if" tone, but the topics are forever things. These are the Step 6 agendas:

a. How soon could we marry?
b. Can we become adults and also please our parents and families?
c. Can we wait to be sexual until we are married?
d. How many children will we have?
e. What kind of birth control will we use in planning them?
f. What are our beliefs and can we synchronize our religious commitments?
g. What are our career plans?
h. What are our education plans? [REVISE to match NEW MAN set here!]
i. Discussing past relationships and killing off the ghosts.
j. Personal or family scandals: Should we share them now or risk finding out later?
k. Reviewing our entire past lives, learning the whole story.
l. Meeting and accepting the whole chain of relatives.

Most marriages which end in divorce have failed because they did not take the time to work through the agendas of Step 6. The super marriages I see, however, inevitably involve couples who took the ultimate risks of knowing: They revealed their worst secrets, fully aware that this knowing could end the relationship. But they also seemed to know, too, that they loved the other person enough to let them know the darkest secret because they believed they would be forgiven and affirmed and valued in spite of the truth.

I said recently to a couple just a month away from their marriage: "You have done your homework. Both of you spontaneously told the secrets of your past lives, bringing in the bulldozer to level the ruins of earlier mistakes. So there are no surprises to explode your trust later on. And the ghosts that might have inhabited those old and shame-filled memories have been exposed. You have listened, forgiven and fully blessed each other. Those old ruins are now compacted into a solid foundation for this new, life-long, exclusive relationship."

Commit or Break Up Now!

I cannot stress too much the importance of these foundation steps. The final one, Step 6, is what I have called "the last exit on the freeway of love." If either person breaks the relationship after Step 6, the result will be "divorce effects." Grief must work its way out of denial, into anger, through bargaining, burrow through depression and finally come to acceptance and hope that there is life after the loss. If anybody quickly starts up a new relationship as a way of self- medicating for the grief of losing someone, you can be sure that the future will be inhabited by the ghost of the lost relationship. This is the divorce effect.

Here is another image I sometimes use: Imagine that the pair bonding steps are markers along the runway as this jumbo jet plane is rumbling along for a take off. "Rotation" occurs as the plane begins to lift off. So your "couple rotation" comes now. At the end of the work you are doing in Step 6 — at the end of this foundation phase of the relationship — Step 7 marks the point of no return. Like the plane which can no longer abort without crashing, so your relationship cannot be abandoned without plunging you down in the flames of deepest grief. There will be no quick recovery, no trip down the runway again for years while you are being redeemed and healed. Both people, and perhaps others, will be injured and the scars can last a lifetime.

It is not surprising that the Romeo and Juliet syndrome has reached epidemic proportions in our time. What the news reports rarely mention is what the communities learn later: The teen suicide was related in some way to a relationship that went bad or to the inability to get the intimacy calendar and the real world calendar to match. Be sure to keep your friends talking if they are hurting from a broken bonding experience.

When pair bonding is kept before public witnesses during these first six steps, and when you have seen the striking quality of your chosen partner when compared to everyone else, you know the choice is both right and final.

The best bonded marriages are those which became "engaged" when the Step 6 work was largely done. You are ready for doing the serious business of putting the final seal on the relationship. This will require substantial private time.

Steps 7 through 12, the last half of the pair bonding steps, require more time away from the crowds of people. Indeed, you will find your preferences have changed radically. Instead of wanting time with the girls regularly, you eagerly invest time with your future husband. Tell your friends to wait, you will return after two or three years into the marriage, and will continue at an adult level the excellent social friendships you established with them during the preteen and junior high years. For now they need to know that you have secrets to tell and secrets to hear and promises to make. Normally, the intensive peer friendships are invested between ages 10 and 15, and the healthy woman takes her skills at friendship, confidentiality, disclosure and honesty into her exclusive, life-long marriage pursuit.

In Chapter Six, we will look at the couple's private and personal agendas. These are the remaining six pair bonding steps and as you complete the tasks they require you will be building that exclusive, life-long marriage.

Chapter Six

The Couple's Private Agenda—Consummating the Bond

In the last chapter I began describing Desmond Morris' "12 steps of pair bonding." I discovered them in his book *Intimate Behavior.* As a zoologist with special interest in how animals mate and raise their young, he includes humans in his "zoo." I don't think he knows that Creation comes from the hand of a God who loves intimacy. He might be surprised, because it's easy to take Morris' 12 steps and put them together with the second chapter of Genesis and the beautifully unfolding set of steps: leaving parents, cleaving or beginning to bond to your partner, then finding yourselves naked together without shame.

Desmond Morris has studied human intimacy and its development mostly because of his interest in how a species survives. He would tell you that if anything ever happens to weaken human pair bonding — the special life-long, exclusive monogamous bond between a man and a woman — the species will be in danger of extinction. It takes about 15 years to launch a healthy kid who can bond and start over in a new exclusive family setting. And if life were simpler, 15-year-olds could marry easily. But from about 13 to 20, most of us need to grind out the complicated skills of dealing with a high-tech, high-priced culture before we marry. We've got to get our bonding right and be ready for marriage, because if bonding breaks down, our kids suffer with us. If they experience abandonment or abuse, their future bonding will likely be damaged, too. Their future sexual behavior is more likely to be promiscuous or rapist or compulsive than if they had come from an exclusive love relationship between father and mother. It is not inevitable, as you will see in Chapter 8, "Coming Back When Things Go Wrong," but across the species or across any human culture, it is easy to see symptoms that pair bonding has been mortally mangled by a lot of folks.

When you look around you or in the mirror, you will be able to name young men and women who are facing this unusual risk. So study this chapter, then stand in front of your own private mirror and have a conversation with yourself. You may even want to have a serious imaginary conversation with the man of your dreams even though you may not have met him yet. Promise him the kind of healthy woman who can form an exclusive, life-long bond. And use your influence among your friends. Ask them questions: "What do you really want for the rest of your life? Do you want exclusive life-long loving or a series of divorces and the lonely life of the singles scene?"

For a Lifetime?

If you want a bond that will last for a lifetime, you can develop a pattern in your search for intimacy that will forever change your behavior. You can choose a courtship and marriage style that matches your instinctual hunger and virtually guarantees that you cannot abandon your spouse and children. Look this over. You may think it is worth taking Desmond Morris' research seriously. Here are some of his purely secular observations:

1. *Make each step in the pair bonding sequence a place to stay awhile.* Move so slowly that you become completely relaxed with intimacy at Step 4, hand-to-hand, before moving to the ecstasy of Step 5, for example, arm-to-shoulder.
2. *Skip no steps.* Pay no attention to TV, to movies or to the fast talk of your friends, who are running all of the pair bonding red lights in order to get the sexual buzz of the later steps. If you skip steps it is like missing key training for an Olympic career. Your bond will be profoundly damaged and is almost sure to break.
3. *Value the people involved.* You have been given this most amazing capacity to form an exclusive bond with *one person*. Fooling around just for kicks would be a little like trashing your own home or torching the sports car of your dreams. The

exception is this: a house or a car can be replaced. There will never be another *you,* or another *him,* and your children will have no second chance for honest and healthy parents. The two of you are *non-renewable resources,* so treat yourselves well.
4. *Avoid spending intimate, extended time kissing* until Step 7. If the lips touch the other person before the work of Step 6 is finished, it is important to keep the kissing at the conventional level. That means, kiss him quickly in arrival or departure rituals, much as you kiss your parents because of their importance to you as their daughter.

In Chapter 5 I outlined the first six steps of pair bonding. You will need to develop these steps in the normal social traffic in which you move as a healthy individual. Keep your circle of friends close while you are locating the man of your dreams and beginning to find out whether the two of you are for keeps.

Now, in this chapter, I want to walk you through the final six steps which will consummate the bond and seal it for a lifetime. Remember that the engagement, plans for a wedding date and synchronizing family connections were all negotiated as a part of Step 6. At Step 6, with all of its candor, shared secrets and serious planning, it was healthy to hear yourself saying, "Here we've been talking like we are getting married, and you haven't formally asked me to marry you."

I cannot stress too much that this "do the work then ask the formal question" is an excellent sequence. It means that nobody is following a cue sheet, but that both of you are following the good, healthy bonding procedures that are written deep in the core of your personalities.

The work of the final six steps is so intensely personal that you will now tend to pull away from the crowd and seek out the privacy you need to complete your exclusive, life-long bonding process. As you sense your need for more private space, keep your hormones and your bonding sequence from running away by doing this:

1. Make a covenant to avoid absolute privacy.
2. Make it a rule that parents and friends do not abandon you and devastate you by creating too much privacy. Announce to them that they are free to walk in any time. This creates a community of family and friends whose casual presence can keep you from rushing these final, slow cementing bonding steps.

3. Plan your time together with intentional and active events.
4. Spend your endless conversation hours with witnesses around you. The shopping mall or the all night restaurant are ideal. In a crowd you can get a complete confidential environment and still have anonymous supervision from the masses around you.

The Pair Bond's Interior Mansion

First touch, hand-to-hand, occurred at Step 3. The physical contact was light in the arm-to-shoulder and arm-to-waist steps, too. Now your couple posture changes. You have been side by side until now, but with Step 7, you turn facing each other:

7. *Face-to-face.* Desmond Morris calls this step "mouth-to-mouth." He uses the title to stress the importance of waiting until the first six steps have been built before engaging in intimate, extended kissing. Morris points out that intimate kissing serves the purpose of "immunization." Benign bacteria from each person's digestive system are exchanged in extended open mouth kissing. This protects you when you visit his tribal headquarters and eat the meals laced with his family's bacteria. Some authorities report that when parents kiss newborns they start up the baby's digestive systems with bacteria compatible to those of the family which will parent the baby.

Desmond Morris' caution is important to you because most teen and young adult bonds today are fatally flawed by premature intimate kissing. Extended couple kissing triggers sexual arousal. Once sexual arousal is experienced, the unfinished work of Steps 1 through 6 tends to be abandoned. If you don't go slowly in the first six steps, a prematurely physical or sexual relationship is almost certain to occur. It will tend to be shallow and deformed because it is stuck at the level of a for-kicks-only friendship. Such a relationship predicts a breakup that is messy and a heartbreak romance in every way. It simply has not built a lifelong bond. But Step 7 in a healthy relationship sets up far more face-to-face intimate behavior than kissing.

Now the couple, with total vulnerability to each other, with childhood and past secrets revealed, can give their eyes to each other. For the rest of your lives, keep this face-to-face inspection time a ritual on a daily basis. No deception, no inappropriate secrecy can survive if the eyes meet and all questions are answered.

Chapter Six: The Couple's Private Agenda

Couples married for 50 years or more typically hold each other at arms' length and study the face in order to draw strength from each others' faces, especially the eyes. If you want to be an honest person, give your husband regular opportunity to look deeply into your eyes. Sit across from him, not beside him, for meals. Turn toward him when he is talking, even if he is talking to the children or to someone else. Watch him with your vulnerable face.

By Step 7 in a relationship, the two know each other so well that they read more from each other's face than from the words. Listen as a nicely bonded, mature couple is talking privately. They rarely need to finish a sentence if they are facing each other. They can read infallibly the message written in the 18 square inches of face which surround the eyes.

Scientists who study the brain-eye-speech connections now are suggesting that we can detect lying by watching specific eye movements in a speaker. Couples have known this for centuries. Parents know it, too. That's why they grabbed you as a little sweetheart, got on their knees and said to you, "Look at me and tell me again what you have been doing!"

But virtually all of the couple's face-to-face time is invested in positive nurturing of each other:

a. Communication, extending the "knowing" boundaries.
b. Receiving energy to build the dream you share.
c. Accepting the assurance that the engagement is, indeed, secure.

Because the first six steps were so well built, Step 7 is a resting place, a secure place, in the sequence. There is less public clinging in the arm-to-waist style. The couple often stands free of each other, enjoys watching each other at a slight distance, even. They are sure of a wedding soon, of promises made to each other, of dreams celebrated and affirmed for each other. Now with all of these life issues settled, it is good to relax and simply be in the other's presence without clinging.

8. *Hand-to-head.* This facing posture goes beyond intimate kissing and non-verbal reading of the eyes. Eventually, the hands will go to the face and head. While talking, reading the eyes and face and bonding to the face, the hands involuntarily play games. With fingers they outline or highlight the facial and head features. Ears, mouth, nose and hair are easily targeted for gestures of caressing touch. These head and face games should be patented. They will be unique to you and your husband-to-be. No one will ever see these salutes you have developed for each other. If, lying recovering on a hospital bed, you were to greet each other with these gestures, other guests would leave the room. We all recognize the private games of hand and face which a couple has developed, even though they were never exactly duplicated in our own repertoire of loving touch.

Hand-to-face touch is often more sexually arousing than kissing, so the agenda is clearly visible now. If the real world calendar for your wedding day is far, far away, you will need to avoid the absolute privacy where intimate gestures are appropriate. Set the rules to synchronize your automatic intimacy needs calendar with the wedding calendar, and keep your intimacy and responsibility integrity-bonded together.

9. *Hand-to-body.* Knowledge of your partner's body increases day by day, and, without your knowing it, you will realize that you have a very complete knowledge of how he occupies space. His shape, his weight distribution, the unique configuration of his fingers, hands and feet — all of these are your domain. You could identify him by any of these parts alone. Desmond Morris stresses that this final step before naked and honest presentation does *not* include genital touch. But now the two of you are care-givers. If there is an injury or pain, each will find the area and give it the healing touch or kiss. There is virtually no holding back because of a sense of impropriety. It is easy to see that the next step will be in the spirit of the oldest love story of all. Let me use honest and parallel terms for the woman and the man in my own translation of Genesis 2:25: "And the man and the woman were both naked and they were unashamed."

The Citadel Chamber: Ultimate Safety

Dozens of times I have heard it: "It was terrible. Everybody said they were doing it, so I found this guy and we had sex. But it was terrible!" There is simply no way for a man and a woman to have super intimacy without investing time in building the whole castle of love. You will see that these final three pair bonding steps can be glorious. But they must be reserved for full trust, legal security,

Chapter Six: The Couple's Private Agenda

public covenant and blessing and patient exploration. Only then will you be sure to find yourselves easily "naked and without shame," in the positive, beautiful imagery of the Judeo-Christian doctrine of Creation.

It is worth sacrificing almost everything else to "get yourselves to the church on time!" It may seem like a big hassle to synchronize the real world calendar and your intimacy needs calendar. But the only adequate foundation for genital contact is a publicly celebrated marriage. Only those conditions provide solid emotional security for each of you and guaranteed proof that you are taking full responsibility for each other, now and forever. Unless you build the castle's citadel as a safe place — private for the two of you but visible to all — insecurity will stalk your lives.

You will hear some talk about "sexual sin." You may hear about "fornication" and "adultery," for example. You can jump ahead to Chapter 9 if you want to get to the root of the issue of sexual sin as the Bible describes it. But it is not as simple as naming sins. Sin is only a theological word meaning "DISASTER." Anything which is destructive is sin. So Chapter 9 is entirely given to walking you through the Bible images and texts which celebrate the marriage and sexual relationship at its highest ecstasy. You will find, if you open your own Bible and follow me through that chapter, that the Bible teachings are positive and true because they accurately describe the way things are! I had a theology teacher in college who used to shock me every time he reminded me of that. He said, "Nothing is true *because it is in the Bible*. It is in the Bible *because it is true!*" So don't imagine that any of your friends are going to escape the tragic consequences of their choices and their behavior simply because they don't know the word sin. They hurt deeper because of their ignorance, and likely don't know how to get their devastation healed.

Now look at those final pair bonding steps which symbolize the best of intimacy:

10. *Mouth-to-breast.* Here is where Desmond Morris gives up. As a zoologist he is baffled. No other species, not even one among the primates, does what the human male does. The human male who began life suckling at Mother's breast, returns now to his wife's breast. It is a gesture of tenderness and trusting dependency, as if to say, *I need you. I draw strength from you. If you love me and believe in me, I can be strong.* So when a man reduces himself to this gesture of absolute weakness and dependency, he is preparing himself for the tenderest experience of his life: sexual union with his wife. Creation's amazing architect designed us so that new life is created only under these conditions of total vulnerability and tenderness. It is easy to see why date rape, violent rape and premature sex for kicks all are really shabby. A baby could be conceived from rape or sex play, but nobody is ready to give it the care it deserves unless they have taken the time and the trouble to create a safe relationship that will create a safe place for the child.

11. *Hand-to-genital.* Speech continues to fade as intimacy increases. The speaking portion of the brain tends to surrender now to the deep and almost instinctive rituals which will consummate the couple's sexual union. To "know" the person ultimately requires the exploration of the source of life and of ultimate pleasure. So the husband and wife admit each other to the most private secret — to know the miraculous genitals with their power for creating life and of giving the highest ecstasy lifelong.

Anyone who seduces a person to gain sexual contact without carefully and slowly building the steps of bonding will be sure to violate the other person, since the automatic physical gestures that move toward intercourse will take over and sex will happen. The result will be date rape, marriage rape or a bad scene which devalues you and your partner. You will have jeopardized your emotions and your healthy sexuality and that of your future spouses and children. Immediately and finally, you will carry a load of guilt, shame and loss.

12. *Genital-to-genital.* Knowing your husband completely and his knowing you symbolizes the giving up of all privacy and secrets. The two are becoming one in every way. You now know each other through the careful building of the steps of intimacy. Penetration and the union of your bodies in sexual intercourse will be the best statement of your affection you have yet made. This ritual of loving will be your special symphony of commitment on your wedding day and for literally thousands of days throughout your marriage.

Risk-Proofing Your Marriage

Your instinctive sense of responsibility has told you to protect your man. You protect him by being honest with him and by keeping your relationship and its health your top priority. But if you want long term risk-proofing for your marriage, here are a couple of bonding tips:

Play all twelve strings on this instrument of life-long loving. Busy couples easily get bogged down with jobs, meals, children, even recreation and moonlighting. But protecting your marital bond requires time for face-to-face, voice-to-voice and hand-to-head exchanges and rituals. You can spot serious defects when the two of you no longer look into each other's face when speaking. The cure requires starting over and playing those early steps as the lower and foundational strings of your instrument of love.

If your lives get busy, schedule time for each other as a top priority each week. A healthy marriage can sustain some spaces in the togetherness, and since a few days apart make you more eager than before to be together, you can literally make up for lost days. Simply book extra time together, a get-away weekend or a special "date." Focus on each other, on listening with your eyes as well as your ears and on stroking face, hair and the body in non-sexual ways. Bonding is mostly communication, the knitting together of mind, affections, beliefs and values. Lifelong, durable bonding takes time. There is no short cut.

In Chapters 5 and 6 I have spread out the story of how two become one — the mystery of pair bonding. It is a beautiful story. And the internal mansion you will build together is more complicated than the visible bonding steps I've described. But only the two of you will be able to describe the texture and the quality of life inside the bond itself. You deserve to tell that story to each other. Your children and grandchildren will thank you for building well.

Chapter Seven

Your Center of Gravity!

My father posed a question for me early one morning. "Did I ever tell you about the day you were conceived?" he asked.

We were milking cows before daylight. I was about your age when he asked that question! I was glad I was hiding behind the flank of the cow when he asked it. He couldn't read the shock on my face.

I cleared my throat trying to hide my nervousness, and managed to respond calmly, "I don't think you ever did."

So he told me. Daddy had to know that I had entered into my visible manhood. I was now slightly taller than he was. After all, I had grown nine inches in height during the last school year. Now this question! Of course, he wasn't dumb. Dad talked to me about everything. He taught me everything he knew. Now, obviously, he was going to teach me something about my sexuality.

In my wildest imagination, I never thought a sex talk would begin like this! He was starting with my own conception — the heart of the sex issue: fertility. A birds and bees talk would have been less threatening — even laughable, considering what I had already discovered. At this point, I had observed the sexual anatomy and behavior of birds, bees, cattle, horses, pigs, sheep and abundant nearby wildlife. I knew about animal reproduction. Daddy was right. It was human sexuality on which I was only vaguely smart and urgently curious.

Fertility

Dad taught me what he knew. And he made it personal. I am still impressed with his teaching ability.

"I thought your mother might never sing again," he began.

She had lost their first pregnancy. Then, two months later, under circumstances he described for me, I was conceived, and Mother was happy again. I was a "wanted child"!

I never told him about another lesson he taught me. That baby who was lost gave up its space to me. There would have been no room in the womb for my conception if that first baby had gone to full term. Their second child wouldn't have been me. The unique genes from sperm and ovum that created me would have been gone, wasted.

Wow! I almost didn't make it on to this planet.

Wow again! I need to live my life thankfully and fully — out of respect to a baby who didn't make it.

Daddy taught me more than I thought possible about sex, fertility and life.

He didn't know then what I have only recently discovered: for every 100 girls who are conceived, 165 boys are conceived, but we lose 59 or 60 of them to miscarriages. Making a baby boy is very complicated because the "morphology" of the young fetus is female. The ovaries have to be relocated as testes. The vaginal lips seal shut leaving a bright red scar on the scrotum holding the testes. And the clitoris becomes the head of the penis. So, making a boy means having to transform and move and fix several things — many of them at about the ninth week. And miscarriages often occur right then. Making a girl is easier, safer and fewer things can go wrong.

A little girl is created in a special way in which her whole life is organized around her fertility. Her breasts as a woman are an important statement about her identity. But her reproductive sexuality is hidden away. She is wonderfully built to conceive and carry a human baby inside her "center of gravity." Her hips, laced with the fatty tissue which stores her estrogens, act as wonderful "ballast" to stabilize her balance, even when carrying that precious cargo. Someone observed that when girls carry their school books, they carry them in front, usually with both hands. Boys, in contrast will manage to hang them over their shoulders, or dangle them by one hand. So center of gravity for a woman seems to point to that marvelous reproductive system she keeps hidden away.

I call it your center of gravity for another reason. "Gravity" not only refers to issues of weight and falling. It is also a word which means "seriousness." Your sexual identity is the most serious truth about you. So your sexuality and your reproductive system are your deepest secrets but your most important identity markers. I want you to take yourself seriously, so give yourself permission to celebrate the good thing God has done in creating you a woman.

Dad accidentally, or on purpose, set me up to respect fertility, to value conception, pregnancy and birth as major wonders of the universe. He never suggested that sex was dangerous, or that fertility could "get me into trouble." His approach to sex education was a gift which set me up for life — in every way. I was impressed. He made it personal, serious and full of unfolding mystery, packaged exclusively for me!

Dad didn't have the technical vocabulary that you and I have when he talked to me about everything sexual. If he had known more, I'm sure he would have found a way to teach me, just as he did, without embarrassing me or violating my privacy. As a teenager, I had some questions about a couple of things. My journey into adult responsibility might have been richer and a bit easier if Dad had known how to describe them. I'm going to try go further than Dad did for me. But you can do an even better job for your children.

What Are Little Girls Made Of?

There is a wonderful story which unfolds during the nine months when a baby is being created. The old nursery rhyme was wrong. Little girls are not always made of "sugar and spice and everything nice," even though you may have thought the poem was right in describing your little brother as made of "sticks and snails and puppy dog tails"! Actually, however, both girls and boys are made of what I call "the Original Adam." If you like this idea, check out a book Robbie and I conspired together called *Lovers: What Ever Happened to Eden?* Like Genesis 2 reveals, everything that is in maleness as well as in femaleness was packed into one person.

Since Adam was split, God has been starting with a "fetal Adam" ever since. We all start out with every thing that goes to make a female and a male. Then, at the ninth week, God "splits the Adam" to make a female or a male. And like Genesis 2, we all seem to be driven for our whole lives knowing that "it is not good" that Adam should be alone, so the hunger for "the other" sends us in search of love and a lifelong pair bond.

All babies develop the same for the first 10 weeks, so far as you can see. If you lost a baby anytime before the 12th week, it would appear to have been a baby girl. Boys and girls look identical as they are developing before that.

At five weeks you can see an open vagina and a pleasure "bump" at the top — obviously the beginning of the clitoris if the baby becomes a girl. But inside the baby there is a pair of ovaries in vertical position, side by side like tiny footballs. They are within the embrace of a "wishbone" made of the two fallopian tubes — called Mullerian ducts at this time. Anyone looking at this internal sex system would identify female parts.

When those gonads that look like ovaries actually lie down horizontally inside the developing baby girl, they will contain a lifetime supply of fertile eggs — called ova. Each ovum is actually a tiny piece of life material handed down only from woman to woman. Each separate egg carries a full ancestral list of mothers, and adds a signature for the developing girl. She will forever be identified as a world-class mother and will leave her marker on every descendant from her body.

The genetic marker is contained in every cell of her children's bodies — literally billions of separate cells, each naming her and all of the child's mothers, all the way back to the beginning of the human species. This record is housed in the floating mitochondrial DNA which surrounds the nucleus of every cell, much as the egg white surrounds the yolk when you break an egg in the frying pan. Recent discoveries have revealed that all humans share the same original mother: Her marker shows up in every living human being's "mother ladder" in that DNA record.

You can read about the powerful "seed of the woman" in the promise to the first mother in Genesis 3:15-20. Study the whole passage in several translations and check the footnotes to see the amazing importance of women in fixing what went wrong in Eden.

As a little boy is formed, those gonads that look like ovaries in the drawing have to be sealed up, moved, and turned into two sperm factories. In response to the XY chromosome code which says "make this one a boy," the gonads are coated with the mother's androgen chemicals. Then they are suctioned, pulled inside the Mullerian ducts and swallowed as they travel down to the outside of the body. There they are clearly testicles and are housed in the lower section of vaginal lip material. This soft, elastic material becomes the scrotum or sac. It will act as the original thermostat, guaranteeing to keep the testicles exactly three degrees cooler than normal body temperature, which is essential for producing mature and fast swimming sperm. And the scrotum is marked by the continuing scar. You have seen the mark on every baby boy whose diaper you have changed. You have noticed the bright red scar running the full length from the rectum, around the scrotum with its former ovaries now in place as testes or testicles. The scar continues up the underside of the penis. It runs as straight as a surgeon's incision, and it seems to divide the boy's scrotum in half, down the center line of his body. The little boy has been "modified" out of the female model and he has scars to prove he made the journey. That scar was sealed by what I call the "glue of God" as the fetal vagina was closed to form the amazing thermostat sac to keep the sperm factory just the right temperature in cold weather and hot, and to wrap the penis in highly expandable material — just like the elastic vaginal lips in a baby girl which may some day enlarge to allow her to give birth to a baby.

Sexual Pleasure

God must have known how tough it is to be human, especially when life isn't easy. Obligations, work and trouble are everywhere. Next to the recharging energy you get from a full night of sleep, your capacity for sexual pleasure is the best renewal gift Creation built into you. And each person is so magnetically made that the best pleasure comes only through the presenting of sexual gifts I described in Chapter Six, where I called that pleasure union "The Citadel Chamber: Ultimate Safety."

It is fairly common for young boys and girls to discover their pleasure center located in the genitals. Many children discover and become fascinated with this self-pleasuring. It is sometimes called masturbation, and in young children most often happens accidentally. A child of only a few months or a few years is surprised and pleased to have discovered the pleasure.

The differences between the pleasure system in males compared to the pleasure system in females is rooted in the ninth to twelfth weeks of fetal development. Boys and girls start out identical in sexual formation. Some marks of that beginning remain in adults. Since the fetus at nine weeks appears to be female, it is not surprising that every boy child carries breasts. Until pubescence, the upper torso of boys and girls looks alike. The boy's body is formed from the female format, as is obvious by that comparison.

The pleasure centers in girls and boys are differentiated profoundly. By the fifteenth week of fetal development the clitoris retreats and is enclosed inside the vaginal lips in the baby girl, but in a boy it enlarges and rises on the clitoral shaft which forms the penis and encloses the urinary tract in the baby boy. So a young girl who discovers the pleasure center in her clitoris may not have a clear sense that she is touching genitals, since the pleasure is not connected to anything visible, or to any other body function. Boys, however, know where the pleasure comes from, because from first toilet training they have been given a name for the penis. The pleasure center at the end of the penile shaft, remember, is the transformed clitoris in the early fetus. But the boy's urination regularly requires handling the penis, so the sensitive pleasure center gets accidentally stimulated very often.

So for boys there is no mystery about where the pleasure comes from. Besides, those powerful sensations are clearly associated with the privacy of the bathroom our parents teach us. Young girls are more likely to pleasure themselves anywhere they happen to be, and seem not to associate it with a need for privacy. Boys, very early, may tend to be more secretive and knowledgeable about sexual things.

Responsible for Pleasure

So welcome to the world of full adult responsibility for fertility and pleasure which are magnificently built in to your center of gravity. As an outsider to the wonderful world of womanhood, but as a grandfather who celebrates both his granddaughters and grandsons as they embrace their maturity, I want to salute you in the early days of your young womanhood and to welcome you to the wonderful world of being female, responsible and mature. And since you will quickly move to full ovulation, you will be responsible for dealing with your fertility and doing that alone.

If you were lucky, you got your parents' help before you hit your first period. It is pretty typical that this bleeding and sometimes aching ritual gets you a new respect around your home. Dads tend to respect their daughter now as a woman, and your parents coach younger sisters and brothers into looking at you in new and respectful ways. Because your fertility is your center of gravity, it is taken more seriously than a boy's arrival at sexual maturity. He is often left wrapped in shame about his exploding fertility, so it is a blessing to be a woman and to have the banners of womanhood unfurled to announce your arrival.

Even in best cases most boys' arrival at manhood — signalled by first ejaculation of sperm material and followed up by occasional or frequent evacuations — is simply ignored in silence. Most young men eventually decide that "God didn't make a mistake" and that they are not created wrong. But the silence which young men could interpret as disapproval or as family embarrassment or shame often leaves its deep wounds in the years from about 12 to 20. As a mother, you can affirm your son's healthy sexual development and not leave him to suffer inappropriate shame alone.

The arrival of your center of gravity with its new adult fertility is an occasion for looking into the mirror and giving yourself special respect. Your sexual gift is your future connection to one exclusive life-long partner — the dream I celebrated with you in Chapter Five. So the years between the arrival of your full adult fertility charge and your wedding day are entirely your responsibility. Here are some pain alternatives and probable consequences as you accept responsibility for your sexual energy and pleasure.

If you reach out or accept sexual connections with anyone before your life-long partner — if you have premarital sex of any kind — your bonding will be vulnerable to three kinds of risks. Each predicts some kind of lifelong pain.

1. If your sexual bonding occurs without taking up full responsibility for one another through legal marriage, you will be developing a pleasure appetite that is disconnected from the real world of work and responsibility. You will be at risk of having an affair that is free of day-by-day responsibility — sex for kicks, not for intimate sharing.

2. If your sexual bonding occurs early and powerfully but you cannot consummate marriage to cement the promises you made in your heart, you are in for the "adultery effect." Adulterating your bonding means that you are at risk of carrying the ghost

of that early serious commitment like a divorce into your future marriage. A sexual relationship needs daily responsible care or it inevitably breaks, so the divorce effect is very predictable.

3. Coming off of either of the first two examples, above, you would be at risk of having a series of sexual partners. If you become quickly sexual with several partners, you are at risk of slipping into the promiscuity pattern in which you and other people reduce yourselves to mere "pieces of meat" looking for pleasure. This may be the most painful of all effects, because promiscuous people feel absolutely worthless and are doomed to loneliness. They cannot maintain any honest and deep relationship across time. Their bonding glue is neutralized and doesn't work after attaching, then ripping loose from so many people so many times.

In the opposite set of cases — if you abstain from sexual contact until marriage — you are also set for pain.

1. If you set your mind to ignore your need for intimacy and to steel yourself against an honest and very deliberate pursuit of a lifelong partner, you risk overprotecting yourself and paying the price of being cold and indifferent to people. The Pharisee syndrome is making harsh judgments against sinners who have sex, and from this high throne becoming cynical and hardened in pride.

2. In the best of all probable worlds, the young woman makes a peaceable covenant between herself and that unknown man in her future to go for sexual intimacy only in marriage. But the waiting, the cycles of hormonal elevation and the worry that you need to compromise to grab somebody quickly before they are all taken can leave you with feelings of anguish and loneliness. "Will I live to see my wedding day?" becomes the primal wail of the healthy, covenant-bound young woman. Religious young women often cry out asking God to delay the Second Coming of Jesus until they can marry and find the intimacy they yearn for. Your center of gravity is a frequent reminder that you were made for love and for mothering. So the waiting turns into a solitary confinement which feels like a prison in which you rot your young vitality away.

If you feel all alone in your struggle, read in 2 Corinthians 12:7-10 about the Apostle Paul's struggle with a "thorn in the flesh." "Three times," he writes, "I pleaded with the Lord to take it away from me. But he said to me, 'My grace is sufficient for you, for my power is made perfect in weakness.'" Don't be surprised if you feel the identical feelings of desperation and loneliness. The private notes and journals of the greatest religious figures reveal struggles with the sexual frustration of their lives.

So there is pain for you either way. But that is God's wonderful way of making you into a moral giant in a few years. Celebrate the good gift of Creation, and cry yourself to sleep alone sometimes. It is a good thing to ask God "Why?!" as you pay the price of waiting.

Look and listen for the pain of your peers who are dealing with the consequences of casual and easy sexual contact. And pray God's grace of ripening wisdom on those who suffer alone and largely in silence, as you do. Rest assured that there are young men who struggle, as you do, and pray God's protecting grace on all of you.

You saw that boys and girls got their sex systems out of the same original "Adam." The "two" were formed out of "one." So when the Jewish and Christian doctrine of Creation says, "The two shall become one flesh," it is easy to see that, sexually, the male is made to complete the female and the female anatomy is the exact "mirror image" of the male. But the differences are so enormous that men need to patiently study women and women need to patiently study men. It will be destructive for either to judge or to try to control the other on the assumption that both are the same. And the worst thing a woman or a man can do in marriage is to try to make over the spouse to be like themselves.

The Female Mind

"The natural state of the human brain is female," I've sometimes said, mostly to get the attention of men and boys. "A woman's brain is wonderfully healthy, while all men suffer from brain damage." Both girls and boys start out with a girl's type brain, with two hemispheres "wired" to communicate feelings to logical reasoning, for example. And a woman is more likely as an adult to be able to put her feelings into words than a man is. The "damage" to boys occurs this way: Between the 16th and 26th weeks of a baby boy's development, his mother's androgens (male hormones) combined with testosterone from his own developing testicles form a frostlike chemical coating on the entire left hemisphere of his brain. The coating is God's way of masculinizing the brain so he can think like a man. Men are able to focus and become single minded, giving intense attention to anything, almost without distraction — something not so easy for women to do. But this "masculinizing" requires killing off about 25 million fiber optics-like connections between the left and the right hemispheres of his brain.

As you may know, the left hemisphere is the speech center and is generally dominant for right-handed people. So picture this: Little boys have lost millions of fiber optics connections between their left-brain speech and their right-brain feelings–emotions–beliefs–images–music needs. Boys and men may have more difficulty than girls and women in putting their right brain perceptions and judgments into words. And when you remember that the left-brain got the hormone coating, you will understand that a boy's speech often arrives more slowly and with more problems. Nine out of ten children in first grade speech therapy are boys.

The baby girl's brain grows freely, normally and simply blossoms wonderfully. There is uninterrupted communication between the right and left hemisphere. "Global thinking" is that wonderful way that girls and women have of taking in all of the data: the rational and the affectional, the logical and the intuitive. You will be able to make decisions which take into account both the logical factors and the people factors. This will mean that as an executive in the work place, you will see the big picture better than most men. And as a wife and mother, you will see the human dimensions along with the right thing issue. For you, a moral decision is one that balances out what is legal with what is true and right and humane. You can see that women have abilities to cope with complicated issues and we very much need them and the perspective they bring in every decision-making group. We need them on committees and boards; we need them to be vocal and influential in politics, in community issues and in the faith community.

Another wonder of brain development is that both boys and girls have been blessed by what is called "the myelinization of the central nervous system." As you hit pubescence, sexual maturity and sexual responsibility are somehow timed to arrive just as the final touches are being placed on this high speed thinking-and-acting gift. You will know that your "myelin sheath" is completed, right up to the correlation fibers of your corpus collossum, when

the following signs appear.
1. You find yourself wondering where you came from, where you are going and what your life is for.
2. You sometimes ask yourself these and other questions as you stand in front of the mirror in the privacy of your bathroom, or when you are all alone anywhere.
3. You are reflective whenever you get quiet. Sometimes you make it a point to be around people because you don't like the negative thoughts you have about yourself if you are alone.
4. You wonder whether anybody out there respects you, whether anyone would love you for a life time, whether God exists and, if so, whether God understands, values and respects you.

These are wonderful and terrible agendas. They mean that you no longer are a little child. Welcome to the world of adult reality, adult responsibilities, adult priorities, and to the maturity you have been yearning for.

Stand Tall!

Your new maturity looks great on you. I couldn't be happier with who you are or with the way you are wearing the crown of your womanhood. You have handled every "developmental task" with honor and distinction. You are competent to deal well with this central task of being yourself in a world gone crazy. Go for it!

Chapter Eight

Coming Back When Things Go Wrong

Jerri is a young mother for whom very few things went right until after she was 20. Her mother resents her to this day, and abused her from her first breath. Jerri wonders whether the shabby treatment was her mother's way of expressing her anger at being pregnant and having to get married. Two more children followed quickly. Then, when Jerri was six years old, her father left. She watched him drive away with scarcely a good-bye. Remembering that day, Jerri thinks that is when she gave up on ever having a normal and happy life.

Dealing with Abuse and Loss

When I met Jerri in her mid-twenties, she had never seen her father again. But she had been used sexually by a neighbor man while she was still a child. When father isn't there, sometimes a predator thinks he can get away with anything. Jerri was pregnant at 16. She wanted to keep the baby, but her relationship with her mother was impossible. So the baby went up for anonymous adoption.

Jerri was sexually active before pubescence and into her adult years. There were always boys who would pay attention to her because she would give them sex. She desperately needed to feel that she was loved, and the sexual closeness gave her at least temporary satisfaction. The line of boys was endless. At 17, Jerri was pregnant again. This time, her mother arranged for her to have an abortion and signed papers allowing the doctor to remove Jerri's uterus — to make certain she would never again be pregnant! Still Jerri's heart cried out "Daddy" day and night.

When Childhood Is Filled with Pain

This chapter will outline three "case" stories, and for each I will describe what went wrong and then suggest a way of coming back to healing and hope.

The first case is that of Jerri, with her painful family losses.

The second case will be that of Lorna, who naïvely and in pursuit of sexual curiosity was blown away by a single afternoon's episode.

A final case will be that of Cherese, who became trapped in sexual conspiracy within her own family.

Grief and Healing for Abuse and Abandonment

Jerri's complicated adult life gave her a full plate of trouble week after week. She was living on her own, the pawn of more than one man, and often reaching out desperately for new men to give her a few hours of affirmation as they used her sexually. It was clear that she would never break her cycle of promiscuity and trouble unless she could deal with her losses. It would be important for her to take the time and to give herself permission to count and grieve for her major life losses. Here are three of them.

1. Jerri's mother was abusive to her daughter from birth. She threw every put-down I have ever heard of into Jerri's face. The lifelong death-wish Jerri's mother had for her rang in her ears every day: "I wish you had never been born!" If abortion had been legal when Jerri was conceived, Jerri knew for certain she would have been aborted. Her mother was still trying to "abort" Jerri as an adult.

2. Jerri's mother's unfinished business became Jerri's, too. Men were the enemy. "They use you and abandon you — so get even with them!" became their prophetic attitude. Jerri lived out the negative expectations, losing every man that approached her. Jerri was amazed when she discovered the connection between her own promiscuity and her mother's emotional violence toward her, which was her mother's way of showing rejection of Jerri's father.

Chapter Eight: Coming Back When Things Go Wrong

3. Jerri's daddy had walked out on her when she was only six years old. Of course, he wasn't leaving Jerri, but the bitter, cynical, biting woman who is her mother. Nevertheless, the naïve egocentrism of every child turns inward to "blame the self" if the parents disappear or if the parents' marriage is lost.

Shortly after I met Jerri, she learned that Daddy was coming back to see his three adult children from his first marriage. I had urged her to get serious about counting up her losses and grieving for the daddy who drove out of her life 20 years before.

The reunion was heavenly to Jerri. Suddenly she discovered why her mother hated her — she was the image of her father, her complexion and eyes identical to his.

Can you feel some of the things Jerri must have been feeling? She had been a scapegoat — taking abuse that she did not deserve. She was abandoned by her father and left with a parent who was full of unrelenting anger. She managed to survive but was profoundly filled with shame, feelings of worthlessness and a desperate need to find a safe place for affirmation.

Counting the Losses

Let me give some basic rules as foundations for the healing strategies I want to offer you. Here are some definitions and guidelines about self-respect or esteem:

1. "Self-concept," "self-respect" and "self-esteem" are tricky terms, because everyone's sense of self worth comes from other people — not from themselves. How a baby is handled, talked to and protected from bad things that happen builds "self value" into the child. Children who begin life in a family where abuse is present receive "no value" messages about themselves. Families which use emotional abuse — sarcasm, name-calling, ridicule and obscenities hurled at each other — are bankrupting each other's self-respect. When an abuser or a screamer uses such words, it is a sure sign that they are calling their victim exactly what they think they themselves are — a zero. Jerri's mother was running on empty, but a little girl could get no handle on dealing with that. She could not be a "mother" to her own mother.

2. Self-worth or self-respect — the "sense of self" — gets its major shape during the early years of life. Adults who have

been secure, respected and treasured by their parents in infancy and early childhood can take abuse as adults without being devastated. "When Charlene swore at me, I thought to myself, 'She is really hurting!'" is the response of a woman who has a healthy sense of self-respect — whose emotional tank is on "full" from a healthy childhood.

3. People with little self-respect will tend to show little respect for other people. They will meet sarcasm with sarcasm, obscenity with obscenity. When there is one devastated person in a family, it is easy for everybody else to dance the dance of mutual devastation. Eventually, everybody is caught spiraling downward into a black hole of worthlessness. You can learn how persons are valued in a family by listening to how family members talk with each other. Learn to listen and to evaluate how each family member responds.

4. People who experience family devastation tend to respond in one of two ways. One group, the honest and reflective ones, tends to suffer from feelings of extreme inferiority. The other troupe turns into con artists; using a compensatory mask, these women skillfully deceive others into thinking they are beautiful, calm and truly feminine.

The women who feel inferior, the first group described in the paragraph above, withdraw and feel worthless. They do not attempt to make friends and drift deeper into isolation. They are likely to be victims of depression, or they will suffer from feelings of shame and be apologetic whenever someone tries to affirm them or be their friend. "Inferiority" is the unspoken middle name of these reflective, devastated women.

The con artist "facade" female is the second possible response to early devastation of self-worth, as mentioned above. These abused women tend to mask the devastation and put on a happy face, often with overdone makeup. They meet the world behind this compensatory false face.

You will not be surprised to learn that "macho" males also develop from this second response. Every macho male who swaggers, threatens, acts cocky and throws his weight around to get what he wants has damaged, low self-respect. His obscenities, his conspicuous consumption of alcohol, drugs and sex are compensatory and are an attempt to mask to his own insecurity and emptiness. He is likely to try to humiliate an honest male. He will use his arsenal of abuse weapons to devastate any healthy male or any honest male who feels inferior. These weapons may consist of name calling, sarcasm or the use of obscenities — even rape of innocent "inferiority" males — probably because the honest and hurt guy reminds the macho male of how damaged he himself is.

The "machisma" female is the woman who hides behind a facade. Such women are abundant in our culture because so many of us have been emotionally abandoned or abused for so much of our early years. Since the macho male and the machisma female both feel like dirt, they are often early victims of sexual exploitation. Once "turned on" sexually, they tend to become promiscuous as they search for the feeling of being loved. Yet they come away from each encounter feeling a little less valuable than before. So their compensatory acts increase as their pain and insecurity grow.

Filling the Cup of Self-Esteem

The quiet and introverted woman is easily depressed and naturally withdraws from people because she feels worthless. Machisma women and macho men keep bumping people away through their harshness. They go through the motions of sexual intimacy, but they are so full of fear and self-protection that they cannot be vulnerable and seem to have no skills for working on making a relationship truly rich and healthy. They are always searching for love, but they are careful to dump friends before they get dumped. If they do not face their emptiness and need for healing, they grow old and are increasingly isolated from everybody. Such men and women simply will not take the risks necessary for establishing long-term friendships or be vulnerable enough to risk being hurt in love and marriage. But if they can ever face the truth about why they "act tough" as a strategy for survival and self-protection, they can be healed of their devastation.

Since self-respect is actually the cup into which we pour the respect we have received from others, healing demands trusting some other people. Most of us arrive at our teen years and our adult careers with some scars on our self-respect. We have had a close brush with abuse or abandonment of some kind. So I am offering here a strategy that all of us need for the rest of our lives, in one degree or another. Here are some steps to take to fill your cup of self-respect:

1. *Give yourself permission to look for a mentor.* A mentor is any person you admire because of his or her gifts, skills and ways of dealing with all of life. At about age 12 or 13 most girls automatically identify additional "models" beyond their parents as they construct their own vision of adulthood. These models tend to be someone such as a teacher, coach, pastor or neighborhood adult. This is true even for children whose parents have been their childhood models. Our parents can bond to us in childhood, and the best parents provide structure and discipline to make us competent and responsible. But we all need an outside mentor to affirm us and set us free. You can see, then, that a mentor can be a lifesaver for kids with devastating family experiences. If a person needs a substitute parent, it will be important to sort out that need and separate it from the "blessing mentor" need. The best surrogate parents come from families you know well where you can be an "added kid" and put yourself into their healthier family life.

2. *Take an hour in the privacy of your room and list the "losses" you feel.* "I felt abused, abandoned or devastated when I . . ." will get you started. "I felt inadequate, inferior or ashamed when . . ." takes you further. "What I need more than anything else is . . ." may wrap up your best hopes. Try giving yourself permission to tell the truth on paper. Then lock it up or carry it in your purse as your own personal life agenda. You are now ready to take the next step.

3. *Be sure that you do not develop a "crush" on your mentor.* The best insurance against confusing your love needs with your needs for a mentor's blessing is to join one or two best friends in a group approach to cultivating the mentor's blessing. Then, ask yourself whether your mentor could handle your life vision and even your dark fears and secrets.

   A good mentor needs to be so strong that you can imagine telling that person your worst secrets, then you can imagine hearing your mentor say, "You're the most courageous person I have ever met." Watch carefully. Read faces, especially eyes, and listen to how the person talks about people who suffer publicly from the feelings you have hidden away inside. Jesus once cautioned: "Don't cast your pearls before swine." He was warning that a dangerous person, like a hungry dumb pig,

Chapter Eight: Coming Back When Things Go Wrong

is likely to "trample your pearl" of suffering, then turn on you and "rip you to shreds." Since you have already suffered enough, you don't need to be ripped to shreds again. Intentionally look for a casual moment to drop the first piece of truth. Give your chosen person a small piece of your pain first, before you risk everything. Can you hear yourself saying to this mentor you have chosen — a teacher, a pastor or some really mature peer —"I've decided to deal with some of my childhood pain before it messes up my whole life"?

4. *After your small circle of confidential friends has established trust and begun to receive the blessing of a mentor, expand your network.* Every healthy and growing person needs a network of honest friendships that are based on absolute respect for each other. When you have the network you need for a lifetime, it will tend to look like this:

   a. You need about five people from your "workplace." This may be school, your job or wherever you invest 40 or 50 hours each week. Again, think of the faces you can trust, the honest people who will encourage you in your journey to healthy adulthood. These confidential friends are likely collected from your workplace world of school and church. But the teen culture often puts pressure on you to neglect the other three dimensions of your network that you also need, which are described below in items b through d.

   b. Your network will include about five people from your immediate family. If you cannot locate five pairs of honest eyes and absolute respect for you among parents, brothers and sisters, you can pick up a few others from the other groups. But promise yourself that your husband and children will be honest, absolutely respectful people. You can then repair this side of your network.

   c. There will also be about five people from your extended family. These are cousins, aunts, uncles and grandparents. Imagine yourself saying to these select relatives the same thing you wanted to say to your admired mentor: "I've been through a lot, but I've decided to face it and get on with being healthy in spite of it." If you cannot identify about five people in this part of your network, look for a way to enlarge one of the other groups.

d. Finally, you will need about five people from your lifelong collection of neighbors, childhood friends and classmates. You need to check them out in the same way you evaluated a potential mentor, slowly revealing your decision to put your pain to rest.

What may surprise you is that nobody can develop an unlimited network of close friends. But each of us needs about 20 friends who really know us and provide unconditional respect for us. We need to keep up-to-date in these friendships. Dr. E. Mansell Pattison described the characteristics of a healthy network of friends:

1. *There is frequent contact* — weekly is best, and face-to-face is better than by letter or phone.
2. *There is a positive emotion at every contact.* You feel suddenly better and healthier, and break into a smile upon sighting each other. Dr. Pattison makes the point that we should not keep people in our networks if they are doing negative things to themselves or to us. It takes too much energy. We may have been stuck with our family during childhood, but we can choose healthy, supportive relationships now that we are becoming adults. Healthy people do not violate, humiliate or berate family members who have abused them, but healthy folks don't continue to dance the dance of abuse either.
3. *There is a risk that the relationship might cost you something.* You might have to interrupt your life to help the person in an emergency.
4. *The risk is mutual.* You know that the people in your network would interrupt their lives to help you in an emergency.

Look at what you have if you intentionally create and maintain a healthy network of friends: If you suffered verbal or physical abuse as a child, if you were abandoned by a parent or if you felt exploited and misunderstood when you were a helpless child whose freedom was very limited, rejoice now! You can now create a network of respect and affirmation, and be "re-parented" and mentored. You can create a new "family" of persons who will give you support and encouragement. And you can give as much as you receive. Health and healing will flourish as we all enter into these intentional networks.

Seduction on a Summer Afternoon

Lorna made her marvelous transition into womanhood earlier than most of her classmates. They seemed so silly and childish. She liked being fully developed, and the time she spent with a mirror paid off in attention from older boys. But Lorna's parents had set a rule: no dating until age 16. And she knew they were serious. So one way to assert herself, she thought, was to hammer away at changing their minds.

It was Bobby who really changed their minds. Not that he phoned or begged. It was just that Bobby was from a family in their church, and they trusted him and his family. "A tennis date?" Lorna's father asked. "Let's not call it a date, and you can go with him for the afternoon. Be home by five o'clock."

Lorna would tell you as she told me: "I don't know why it was so important to go out with Bobby. I liked him, but I didn't really know him very well. We never played tennis. He took me for a drive and told me how special I was to him. I needed to hear that, I guess. We all do. While he talked he pulled me closer and closer. He told me right out, 'I want to have sex with you. Nobody will be hurt by it because nobody will know. OK?' I had been rebelling against my folks about not letting me date, so I said, 'I don't know whether we should.' "

The scenario was pretty typical. She was curious and rebellious; he knew exactly what he wanted. He took charge by telling her what she wanted to hear. She was compliant, partly because she thought women do what their men want them to do, but also because she wanted to be sure Bobby would keep on liking her. Whatever Bobby wanted, he got. He knew the lines to lead a girl into bed. He was accustomed to being a winner. This all too typical scenario is date rape, even though Lorna passively consented.

When she returned home, Lorna was shattered. She burst into tears. In a few minutes she blurted out what had happened. There was a face-off between fathers. Lorna was humiliated twice: once by Bobby and now by the open warfare between two families who had been friends. The sex episode exposed the news of the most embarrassing humiliation of her lifetime.

You won't be surprised at any of the effects which showed up immediately:

1. Bobby said she was "trash," and that he "would never go out with her again if she were the last woman on earth."
2. Lorna was mysteriously attached to Bobby. She wanted more than anything to be with him. She was bonded to an abusive and seductive young man.
3. In her embarrassment, Lorna changed. She masked her shame and at the same time found that many other boys were looking her over. She didn't know whether all of them knew of Bobby's date rape, but she began to dress differently. Her new heavier makeup and more provocative clothes got her more and more attention. She was a civil war on the inside. She felt like trash! But she liked the attention that came with her new status, since it gave her temporary relief from the humiliation and shame that plagued her day and night.

Sanctifying Sexual Energy

Lorna was reduced to a sex object. Bobby trashed her suddenly in an afternoon when life ended on this planet for her in any recognizable form. If she cannot unravel that sex episode on a sunny afternoon and let go of it, it can easily control the rest of her life. She can develop an appetite for Bobby or for any other "Bobby" and feel in her desperation that "any Bobby" will do, if she can only get a temporary release from the vacuum the last guy left. This triggering of high sexual appetite is common with victims of emotional rape and of either women or men who are used and then abandoned. Their high speed sexual chasing turns out to be what we now call "sexual addiction" or "fatal attraction."

Here are some of the universal effects on a person who has been reduced to a sex object:

1. Lorna began to lose her sense of self-worth and to think instead of her "sex worth." How much pleasure can she get, how soon, how often? What strategies can she use to get the most, quickest, with new dimensions and limited attachment?
2. As Lorna became preoccupied with sex and found that she needed sexual contact to feel worth anything, she started seeing other people only as "meat." They became objects, were held at arms length, never to be trusted and loved "subjectively." Her sexual yearning tends to also be "objectified" — made "external" to her real self.

Chapter Eight: Coming Back When Things Go Wrong

3. Lorna has become a sex addict. She may be a sexual fantasy and masturbation addict, or she may become a "user" addict. This compulsive sexual rampage she is on will make sexual contact less and less satisfying as she tries to silence her deep sexual yearnings by exploiting more and more partners.

You can identify sex addicts by the way they use people and then dispose of them before it costs anything permanent. Addicts feel ashamed when an episode is over, whether it is masturbation or sex with someone else. They feel "less a person" than before. But after a few hours or days or weeks, their desire awakens. They slip into a sort of hypnotic trance and begin again the ritual that is calculated to deliver the next episode of pleasure. Then they hit shame again and the cycle is complete. The addict's cycle goes round and round as she digs herself a black hole of shame. While she was falling in love with Bobby, Lorna was innocent, wholesome and at ease with almost anyone. Now that she has been devastated she has begun to "signal" men everywhere that she is devastated and also available. Her sexual episodes began on that summer afternoon, and she wonders whether she can ever get them to stop.

Recovering from Sexual Addiction

Sex addicts, by this definition, require healing for self-respect. They, like Jerri with her early family disturbance, will keep slipping into the black hole of self-contempt, and will feel like dirt. Those are "shame" feelings. Shame feels worthless, dirty, incompetent. Shame makes you feel like you are a fraud: *If people knew what kind of a rotten person I really am, they wouldn't want anything to do with me.*

So healing from compulsive sexual behavior requires outside help — the confidential network, the mentor to whom you can reveal the best and the worst about yourself, and the extended support network I outlined earlier in this chapter.

But "sexaholic" addiction requires special help — healing of core ideas about yourself and your sexual energy. In some ways the sexaholic is like the foodaholic. Eating disorders are another compulsive behavior that points to serious self-esteem problems. We are glad that alcoholics can "swear off" alcohol and abstain for the rest of their lives. Foodaholics and sexaholics can't do that.

Sexaholics need affirmation and love to survive, even though they have hardened themselves against vulnerability and "subjective" intimacy. The shame-based sexaholic must continue to be a sexual person and must deal with sexual thoughts, issues and energies day by day. What the sexual addict must find is a way to *transform* sexual ideas and practices. Here are some strategies to help work toward that transformation:

1. *Get serious about understanding sex.* A good place to begin is Chapter 9: "Take Your Curiosity to the Bible." If you have a research interest, don't be afraid to read the technical journals and research books about human sexuality. If your pastor or other respected mentor or surrogate parent can be trusted with your curiosity, ask to borrow the best books they have or find out where to go for information. Your "center of gravity" is so urgent with its powerful sexual energy that you simply cannot abstain from thinking about sex. You may succeed for a few weeks, but denial soon explodes from underground. When it explodes, your compulsive sexual behavior is likely to set a world record that drives you deeper into your shame pit. So get good, honest, technically accurate information. You can find more about this from me in my books *Bonding: Relationships in the Image of God*; *Re-Bonding: Preventing and Restoring Damaged Relationships*; *Lovers: Whatever Happened to Eden?* and *Parents, Kids, and Sexual Integrity.*

2. *Focus your imagination on what you really want.* Sexual imagination is controllable — like making your own images to watch. If some compulsive sex imagination strikes you, be ready with some mental videotape of your sexual future as you *want it to be*. If you fill that video with explicit images of your "exclusive, lifelong intimate knowing" of a partner, then you are rehearsing fidelity, monogamy and intimacy as you think sexually. When some inappropriate image appears, you can quickly transform the person or people involved into *imagining their best future in exclusive, lifelong intimate bonding* in their own marriages.

Since your sexual energy is so persistent, you have a lifetime discipline job on your hands. But, as all of us know, wonderful possibilities always show up alongside terrible potential risks. So accept the challenge of surrendering your sexual energy to God and

Chapter Eight: Coming Back When Things Go Wrong

accepting *sanctifying grace* day by day to keep you on the track of fulfilling your best dreams. And don't worry about dreams that occur when you are in deep sleep. Most of these we do not remember, thankfully! But dreams which are interrupted by your awaking are often remembered. Remember that most of what you dream is garbage which your deep consciousness is disposing of. So let the stuff go. People who have been deeply hurt or experience painful family stress often have nightmares. Sometimes these disturbing dreams are violent and frightening. But if these are really garbage disposal dreams, you are wonderfully and unconsciously letting go of the junk which has been messing you up. So a garbage dream episode might just be some necessary housecleaning.

Caught in the Family Nest!

A final case will be that of Cherese, who became trapped in sexual conspiracy within her own family. Until she was 24 she blamed herself. Her father put a sexual move on her when she was 12 years old. Her older brother and mother were at the mall, and in a rare occasion when only Cherese and her dad were at home he began touching her breasts. Then he actually forced her to do sexual things for him. Last of all he warned her that she was only a little girl and threatened, "Don't imagine anybody will believe you if you tell them what happened. I'll just say it never happened and what will you look like then? Everybody will know you are lying."

Cherese was terrified, humiliated, frightened and felt like her life was over. Everything at home changed from that moment on. If it ever looked like she would be left alone in the house when her father might appear, she would panic. She begged not to be left alone. Her mother wondered what could be wrong with her. She would cry and beg to go shopping, go to church, anywhere rather than stay at the house. But she could never tell the truth. Occasionally it happened again, then again. Now it was predictable that there would be sex with father every time he could find her alone or manage to take her alone in the car on some pretense.

When Cherese began to fill out her adult body, it kept happening. She gained more than 50 pounds the year she turned 13. By the end of high school she had topped 200. Her father mocked his "fat girl," and her mother was enraged that she was always gorging on food. When she was a sophomore, at 15, her brother and two of his friends trapped her and raped her in her brother's bedroom when their parents were out for the evening. She turned up pregnant after that orgy, and her brother made a big deal of arranging for the abortion and threatening to tell Mother that she had been fooling around with boys from school. Nobody would believe her story, he reminded her.

How Victims Survive

A girl needs her father's affirmation, his protection and his attention in every possible way if she is to learn to trust a man for a lifetime. Since fathers represent God in some mysterious way, girls who are father's victims tend to lose even that final desperate sense of trust — the ability to believe that God is there for them.

So survival for victims of father incest is grim. Stripped of a ground for faith in miracles of grace and forgiveness, they often feel more alone than any other victims in the world. And at the day-to-day level, they absolutely do not trust men, no men of any kind anywhere.

Cherese had dropped out of music and athletics, but she kept up her art classes during high school. It was never clear what prompted her teacher to pay attention to Cherese, but during her senior year, the teacher invited her to lunch, then to an overnight stay, then to move in after graduation. So out of father and brother incest and abuse, Cherese was vulnerable to falling into a lesbian love-crush with the adult woman mentor.

Girls and women who have been victims of male abuse deserve top notch therapy to get a perspective on how the abuse may have warped their view of life and of men. The three times an abused woman needs professional therapy are (1) immediately following the abuse, (2) as they approach marriage, and (3) at the time their own children approach the age at which they themselves were abused.

Without healing in feelings and attitudes toward men, victims of incest may find relief in friendships, even intimacy, with a woman or with women. But they have not found a healing cure. Cherese continued to carry a hundred pounds of weight as her shame baggage. Her healing will have to follow the pattern of Lorna, the compulsive sexual addict. The compulsive eating and now her abandoning of the vision of love and marriage are driven by devastated self-esteem, anger at all men and a determination to retaliate for a lifetime.

Dancing with a Domineering Stressor

What I have described in Cherese's family is a "Stressor Family." There is a dominant stress maker, usually her Dad but sometimes her abusive brother. Cherese knows that when she is likely to have to deal with either of them alone in the house, she must be on her guard. She hides her own needs and feelings, because Dad or brother has moved in like a snowplow, and the man's agenda is the only agenda. Cherese's mother, as well as Cherese herself, are sometimes called "co-dependents;" they are caught in a dance over which they have almost no control. Often these co-dependent dancers never get their needs met. They may be called obscene names or assign such names to themselves. They feel bankrupt. They have no rights, feelings or respect. They are unable to tap the family's emotional resources to nurture them. They are easy victims of compulsive, almost unexplainable exaggerated emotions and behavior. A victim is "co-dependent" because they are helping to perpetuate the conspiracy by their shame-based continuing participation in the destructive behavior.

The stressor may be any member of the family. That person may suffer a serious or terminal illness which demands everybody's first attention. Or it may be an imagined or fake illness. It may be a food addiction, workaholism, alcoholism, a rage addiction, gambling or sexual promiscuity. It may be addiction to religion, community volunteering or any emotional or humanitarian compulsion which makes the family pay the rent for the endless hours the stressor spends attacking, abandoning or abusing the family.

Escaping Crazymaking

Co-dependency is tough to break. How do you break away from this dance of deformity? How do you discover who you might really be if you were taken seriously, valued and nurtured into responsible adulthood?

Here, again, the help is outside the family. The rule is simple: Find health somewhere else and get yourself emotionally adopted into a set of relationships where everybody counts, and everybody is valued and respected. You can find families like this if you will connect with church, scouts or community recreation, and keep your eyes and ears open at school and in the community. You are smart enough, if you are in a crazy-making, stressor home, to spot dangerous people in anybody's house. Here are some tips for locating a healthy family:

1. Listen to how the kids talk about each parent. Ask questions about how they get along with each parent.
2. Listen to how these friends of yours talk about brothers and sisters. Is there an instinct to protect each other?
3. Get yourself invited to stay overnight or to go on a day trip with the family you are admiring. Seeing families interact over a period of 24 hours or more is like looking through a microscope: The real personalities start coming out under normal family pressures.
4. If you can't locate a family with kids your age, conspire with two or three confidential friends to locate a mentor with whom you can open up your highest hopes and deepest hungers and needs. Follow the suggestions for finding a mentor given earlier in this chapter.

You are rebuilding a sense of your own worth, so pay attention to your networking and truth-telling as discussed in this chapter.

When Victims Marry

Occasionally a victim of incest or family rape marries, often to escape the obscenity of being forced to have sex with a family member or a relative. Since these victims are devastated and feel like dirt, they frequently become seductive and sexual with a relatively innocent young man. Once married, the sexual activity typically becomes unbearable or repulsive. The boundaries that were broken by a father or a brother or a cousin are now rebuilt to keep a husband away.

The marriage may be fatally flawed, unless both the victim and her husband find professional therapy and a community of hope and healing in a congregation or a competently-led 12-step group.

The Bottom Line

It is as simple as this. If you can name your pain, you can be healed of it. In the stories of Jerri, Lorna and Cherese I have wanted to open the basic doors through which many hurting young women may need to walk.

God, who made all things whole, complete and "good," can make you new again. Jesus is the advertisement, the pointer. His abuse, death and resurrection are the "rent" paid to transform you in this present life. In my book *Re-Bonding: Preventing and Restoring Damaged Relationships* I trace the fact that you can become whole and virginal again, no matter what your losses have been. God promised this for his damaged and compulsive bride Israel.

And I am here for you. Heather, Jami and Lesli, you will always know how to find me. But for a thousand other young women, for the rest of my life, I will keep an open line for you at 859-858-3817. Or write a letter to me and mail it to the publisher whose address is in the front of this book. Get your encouragement from any safe person near you, of course, but know that nothing that has happened *to* you needs to *control* you.

Chapter Nine

Take Your Curiosity to the Bible

When I was in the eighth grade, Jim Deaver, Ed Zortman, Lyman Dewell and I used our spare time trekking to the back of the classroom to consult the *Webster's Unabridged Dictionary*. Bruce Ramsay, our teacher and the principal of the Fowler Elementary School, thought we were energetic and bright boys. Actually we were often searching for technical terms about human sexuality. We were learning, by the not-so-innocent age of 13, a lot of *non*technical sexual words. We suspected that if we could find them, there were powerful, plain English words that were not violent and obscene. We had a little luck, and found our vocabularies growing. We didn't pronounce all of the words right, since the silent dictionary wasn't much help to farm boys who had never heard most of those excellent English words about sexual matters.

I was lucky in my search for understanding the meaning of being human and sexual, since my search also went to church. I was inducted at about 13 into the youth group. I am thankful for all the affirmation I got at church, and for the way my advisors and teachers showed me how to open up the Bible. My sexual curiosity was blown away by how much the Bible talks about the things I was interested in at age 13.

This chapter offers a walking tour of the Old and New Testaments. Sometimes I suggest a specific version, but most of the time any Bible version or translation will get you to the right stuff.

What I predict is this: *You are going to find, as I did then and as I do now, that the Bible is powerfully positive about your iden-*

tity and about human sexuality in particular. If you find a "sex-negative" statement, look carefully. I have never found a sex-negative Bible statement that was not protecting the crown jewels of human life — personal identity and relationships. I'm inviting you to fasten your seat belt and get ready for *a sex-positive tour of Holy Scripture.*

Creation and the "Image of God"

You are at the peak of God's creation work. In sequence, humans appeared last on this planet. But in responsibility, humans are fixed at the center — responsible for themselves and for the careful management of all animals, birds, reptiles and the earth itself.

The Bible's view of you is that you are the best there is: "Very good!" God said. Which means, "I can't improve on this species, or create one any more complete, competent and full of potential for everything needed on planet Earth."

And the Bible's picture of you is that you are "created in the image of God." Think of what this may mean:

1. Since God is creative, you are born to be creative, and God has shared the gift of sexual reproduction as part of your "creativity."

2. Since God resides in Holy Trinity — Father, Son and Holy Spirit — you will have a yearning to find a place in a Holy Community. You will feel a need to be part of an intimate marriage and family. And since the Holy Trinity exists as co-eternal, co-regent, dialogic unity, so also you will be pained unless your love and marriage and family relationships have "Trinity-like" characteristics of mutual respect and solid unity. Evidently girls and women are highly gifted with this sense of need for relational integrity, for participative intimacy and for keeping all relationships harmonious as long as they live.

3. Since God is just, you instinctively cry out, "No fair!" when you are cheated, and you step in to interfere when somebody else is violated. Evidently boys and men are given a major dose of this side of the image, and most of them are eager to respond to injustice, to cry "Foul!" and to lay down their lives to protect or put right any wrong done to anyone of importance to them.

Chapter Nine: Take Your Curiosity to the Bible 99

4. God's image stamped into your genes means you are uniquely self-conscious, reflective and imaginative. All of the things God is, you are created to reflect.

Now for the sexual part. By some fantastic mystery, God's image in you, the Bible teaches, is expressed in your female sexual system, your identity and everything feminine about you! Let me take the masculine generic pronouns out, using my own translation of Genesis 1:27: "So God created the Adam in God's own image. In the image of God, the Adam was created. Male and female, God created them — from the Adam." You can read almost exactly the same summary in Genesis 5:1-2, where the New International Version of the Bible speaks of Adam in the same way. Check the footnote to see that "man" is actually "Adam." So when they were created, he called them "Adam." Look at the exact sequence of the statement about the man and the woman being created in God's "image." There is something about your being female and feminine that uniquely represents something about God — just as there is something unique about a woman's ability to represent God.

Phyllis Trible, in her amazing book *God and the Rhetoric of Sexuality*, points out that the Old Testament word for "compassion" which describes God's care for us is actually the word for the "contraction of the uterus" as the nursing mother gives her attention to her newborn's survival. That word is used of the real mother when Solomon offers to split the living baby in half in order to settle a squabble between two mothers after one newborn baby was smothered during the night. He knew the real mother would give up and let the baby live rather than have it divided: She was moved with "compassion." God is like that — like a mother who truly loves her own baby. That is one example of how a woman expresses the image of God.

I suspect this "image of God male and female" design means we need to keep a sex-balance everywhere: in marriage, in family, in organizations, in the church — in all of our systems and structures. If God depends on men and women to carry unique parts of the image of God, then we surely don't want to make big decisions without getting both male and female perspectives.

The most amazing sexual mystery is this: God evidently was most happy about how much fun it was to create human beings. If so, we can understand that God's gift of sexuality equips *us* to be creators, too. It takes one adult man and one adult woman to make a baby. We can create more humans! But we are not like some of the species in which one parent can make a baby and take good care of it. The infant-dependent period for humans is very long — about 15 years! Every human baby needs both sides of God's caring "image" to shape it into a healthy adult male or female over at least that long a span of years. Besides having a long childhood, humans need very complicated parenting, requiring specific things fathers do better than mothers and others that mothers do better than fathers. So every baby deserves to have a father and a mother: both sides of that amazing "image of God." And you can look back at Chapter 8 to review the kinds of deficits any kid may have to deal with if that ideal "image bearer" arrangement has been violated or destroyed.

Now, hang on! Being created "in the image of God" seems also to mean that it's "godly" for males and females to long for each other! Get this: the mystery of the Trinity means that God, Christ and the Holy Spirit live in perfect community with each other. Furthermore, Jesus' prayer in John 17:20-23 shows that he yearns to bring *us* into the kind of unity the Trinity enjoys. The Old Testament illustrates this by speaking of God as the "Husband" and Israel as his "Bride." And in the New Testament Jesus is the "Groom" and "head," while believers — the Church — are the "bride" and the "Body." All this leads to a fascinating question: *Is God's "image" reflected in the way we yearn for each other "as a bride for a groom and a groom for a bride?"*

This intimate language also tells us that our need to be united with God's purposes and character, to be holy and fired with justice and compassion, are so deep that God uses almost explicit sexual images to remind us of our need to join purposes with God. Our deep longing to become one with that "other self" — and our need for life-long fidelity to that husband — are God's image in us. But these human, physical yearnings may also be God's way of hooking us — reminding us that human intimacy is only rehearsal for the ultimate intimacy we are working on: intimacy with God.

You can read about the image of God, male and female, in Genesis 1:26-28. Adam was "split" in Genesis 2 into the first man, *Ish* and the first woman, *Ishah*. The man turned against the woman, dominating her, and renaming her "Eve." To read more

Chapter Nine: Take Your Curiosity to the Bible

about this, follow the text and center column words in the New American Standard Bible. Also check footnote "g" early in Chapter 5 of Genesis in many editions of the New International Version Bible. If you get a copy of *Lovers: What Ever Happened to Eden?* which Robbie and I wrote to unravel this image of God, male and female issue, we will walk you through all of these images in slow motion.

But it is equally tragic that "Eve" renamed her husband. He ceased to be *Ish* and she began calling him *Baal.* You can read God's repudiation of that name in Hosea 2:16. There, speaking of his longing for Israel to return from her broken and prostituting ways, God says, "... it shall be in that day, says the Lord, that you will call me *Ishi;* and shall call me no more *Baali."* Your King James Bible carries those contrasting words still in Hebrew. And Israeli women today still call their husbands "Baal," with all of its idolatry symbolism.

When failure damaged the original marriage, God warned the woman: "Your desire will be to your husband, and he will rule over you." You can read that whole tragic story in Genesis 3. Today's woman tends, like the original Eve, to love too much, be too dependent, often demanding that her man be "God" to her — making him a Baal-idol. Many women tend to give up on being strong, whole and high achievers, afraid to compete with the men they need so much. But every healthy woman turns to God as her ultimate refuge and strength, setting her husband free to be *Ish* — her "other self."

The strong, complementary woman is pictured throughout the majestic tribute to women in Proverbs 31:10-31: "Who can find a virtuous woman . . . ?" is the introduction to a grand woman! And look at the ancient epic drama we call the book of Job. In his final chapter, that remarkable and wise old man of God did what none of the line of Old Testament patriarchs evidently did: He granted an equal inheritance to his daughters and his sons. Look at that remarkable statement in Job 42:15.

Man and Woman as "One Flesh, Naked and Unashamed!"

You can see that Adam in Genesis 1 is plural — humankind! "Male and female he created them." Then, Genesis 2 describes how this complete Adam is actually divided to create woman, then man. I sometimes refer to this as "God's first splitting of the Adam!" The text tells us that God created Adam from *'a-dam-ah* — a Hebrew word describing the dust particles of the earth which became the raw materials for "Adam."

When Adam is split into female and male parts of God's image, God is portrayed as a surgeon. Adam's thoracic cavity or rib cage is laid wide open. That cage has ribs (Hebrew *tsela*) so a boat construction word is used. Human ribs like the ribs of a wooden hull of a boat hull support the outer "skin" or covering. When Genesis was translated into the first Greek Bible, the translators called the ribs *pleura*, denoting the cavity where you may have felt sharp pains we still call "pleurisy" — shooting around the entire rib cage.

With this complete Adam laid wide open, God built up the woman from those parts taken from the thoracic cavity, closing up the "Adam body" from which they were taken. These "better parts," we say, "were formed into woman — the feelings, the tenderness for people, the ability to speak her feelings were given to her." You have likely heard your dad or grandpa refer to your mom or grandma as "my better half!" After all, the left-over part of the Adam was the male.

The surgical picture is used to tell us three things:

1. Both male and female are made from Adam, and they are created as temples of the "breath of God" or the Holy Spirit and as bearers of God's image.

2. Sex differences are profound. Women are super-built for attachment and concern for relationships. Men are under-equipped for expressing feelings, but super-built with muscle, strength and the ability to zero in on urgent tasks that have to be done in spite of feelings.

3. Either is incomplete without the other. They were formed first as one; when separated they are alone and yearn for missing dimensions they cannot always identify. The loneliness in the solitary male or female is often felt as a cosmic loneliness. It is not specifically sexual loneliness, but people who run only with their own gender tend to be trying to clap with one hand in a universe which is calling them to a standing ovation.

Chapter Nine: Take Your Curiosity to the Bible

Back to our story: Upon recovery from their surgery, *Ish* and *Ishah* are magnetically attracted to each other. "Wow!" the male said, "this is bone of my bone and flesh of my flesh! This shall be called *Ishah*, for she was formed out of *Ish!*" So there in the presence of God and without a priest, preacher or rabbi, the whole universe cried out: "Because of how they are created, *Ish* shall magnetically bond to *Ishah* and they shall become one intimate flesh, naked and without shame!" Much later, trying to get us back to this wonderful picture of the way it is supposed to be, Jesus added another powerful line recorded for all time in Matthew 19:4-6: "What therefore God has glued together let no one anywhere, anytime, on earth break apart!" These are my loose, but faithful conceptual translations.

I suggest that you work slowly through Genesis 2 in two or three translations and review our unraveling of this chapter in *Lovers: What Ever Happened to Eden?* You can read Jesus' words about the "epoxy glue" bond in Matthew 19 where he is shutting down people who trivialize marriage and recommend divorce for a thousand irrelevant reasons.

Intimate "Knowing," Intercourse, Conception and Birth

I was baffled when I was young because of the way the Old Testament talks about couples and how they get a baby. After a conception, the Bible would say, over and over again: "Adam knew Eve his wife, and she conceived...," "Cain knew his wife, and she conceived...," "Elkanah knew Hannah his wife...." And when Mary and Joseph discovered she was pregnant with the special conception that gave us Jesus, the Son of God, the text reports, "Joseph knew her not, until she had borne a son." You can see this strange language of the old King James Version if you look at Genesis 4:1, 17, 25; 1 Samuel 1:19; and Matthew 1:25. Newer translations are more clearly sexual. Joseph, for example, "had no union with" Mary until she had delivered her son, according to the New International Version.

The Hebrew word translated "know" or "knew" suggests *real* knowing — stripping away masks and secrets. In a healthy, bonded marriage when two people have voluntarily shared their vision and their secrets, they are certainly on the way to "knowing" each other. So the Hebrew idea suggests that an enduring, life-long relationship requires "getting to know" each other, and guarantees intimate joining, union and the literal merging of the two.

The Taboos: Adulterating, Fornicating and Raping

In the Bible there are a few cases where "knowing" is used in the sense of ripping away the secrets and violating a person. One tragic example of this kind of "knowing" appears in Judges 19:25. A man's concubine had left him and was either practicing prostitution or at least sleeping around with other men back in her home town. So he went after her to bring her back. While they were spending the night on the road home, they prepared to spend the night on the streets of Gibeah. But an old man urged them,

> "Let me supply whatever you need. Only don't spend the night in the square." So he took him into his house and fed his donkeys. After they had washed their feet, they had something to eat and drink.
> While they were enjoying themselves, some of the wicked men of the city surrounded the house. Pounding on the door, they shouted to the old man who owned the house, "Bring out the man who came to your house so we can have sex with him."
> The owner of the house went outside and said to them, "No, my friends, don't be so vile. Since this man is my guest, don't do this disgraceful thing. Look, here is my virgin daughter, and his concubine. I will bring them out to you now, and you can use them and do to them whatever you wish. But to this man, don't do such a disgraceful thing."
> But the men would not listen to him. So the man took his concubine and sent her outside to them, and they raped her and abused her throughout the night, and at dawn they let her go. At daybreak the woman went back to the house where her master was staying, fell down at the door and lay there until daylight.

You can read the whole horror story in Judges 19. I have quoted the New International Version of verses 20-26.

When the man found his concubine unconscious on the doorstep the next morning, the man put her on his donkey and took her home. What he did next may have been a parable or merely a deeper sign of his own wickedness. He cut her into twelve parts and distributed her body into all twelve tribal areas of Israel. So the

Chapter Nine: Take Your Curiosity to the Bible

story provoked people to cry out everywhere: "Such a thing has never been seen or done, not since the day the Israelites came up out of Egypt. Think about it! Consider it! Tell us what to do!"

The whole story describes the worst end of the range of things men are capable of doing to women. Since the tragedy of sin recorded in Genesis 3, men have a tendency to regard women as their property and to control them. *That is not God's design or God's will, and men who use women are always under God's judgment.* This story about violent "knowing" is as bad as it gets.

There are other words of illegal and inappropriate sexual contact. The heat of sexual desire sometimes drives people over the edge, with a sort of simple animal passion. "Lie with me" is a King James translation of the use of sexual passion purely for selfish gratification. Joseph, a trusted employee in the house of the Egyptian Potiphar, was propositioned for sex by Potiphar's wife. She "caught him by his garment, saying, 'Lie with me.'" The word for this sexual passion was very much like our use of the phrase, "go to bed," when it means simply "I want your sex, not life-long responsibility and care for you." You can read this story in Genesis 39. Nothing much has changed about being at risk for sexual seduction and entrapment, even today.

A third word in the Old Testament was used to describe sexual seduction. It was a violent term meaning the same as "rape." One of the most tragic stories in the Bible is of the rape of Tamar by her half-brother Amnon. You can read the story in 2 Samuel 13. Amnon devised a plot to trick Tamar, pretending he was sick. Then he begged her to "lie with him," the seductive ploy for getting sex. When she agreed to marry him, but not to play around with him, he forced her to have sex with him; he raped her. Date rape, acquaintance rape and violent rape by a stranger are similar to Amnon's sin against Tamar. You can read the text and see the humiliation Tamar felt, and the vengeance her full brother, Absalom, planned against Amnon. It is easy to see that everything goes wrong when anyone is obsessed with getting sex without responsibility and respect for themselves and the other person.

If you want to work through a terrifying chapter of warnings, most of them calling for the death penalty, look at Deuteronomy 22. When I first read it, I thought it was about premarital sex. But as I studied it, it became clear that this is not about premature bonding, but about one person "using" another sexually. And when you look at how emotionally damaged people are who use other people or get used by them, you may understand a primitive society which said simply, "Kill them!" They had no rehabilitation programs or psychiatrists. And they didn't have Jesus hanging on a cross and rising from the dead to establish a way to be "made new" again. So, damaged people were like broken-legged race horses. They simply had to be killed.

Song of Solomon: Images of Sexual Loving

The classic love song of all time is in the Bible book called Song of Songs or Song of Solomon. Theologians have squeezed the book to try to extract spiritual messages, but it can be read simply as a book about sexual intimacy. What we have to remember, however, is that sexual intimacy, even holy sexual passion for an exclusive, life-long partner, is the best human picture of powerful faith in God. And when we want to talk about our faith in God, we borrow words from marriage. "Faithfulness" and "fidelity," for example, create images of sexual faithfulness and exclusive marital fidelity. If you want to sample the Song of Songs, try reading chapters 2, 4 and 5. You will see in 2:6 the description of the posture for sexual intimacy. All of chapter 4 describes the yearning of the man for the woman, and all of chapter 5 describes the yearning of the woman for the man. Evidently the "garden" and the "fountain" references are to the intimate genital gifts they presented to each other.

Jesus: Ultimate Respect for Human Sexuality

You can read the highest respect for human sexuality and marriage in the words and actions of Jesus. He says, in a faithful paraphrase: "What God joins together sexually, be careful not to rip apart!" Jesus announces the warning in the face of easy divorce in his teaching recorded in Matthew 19. He restates the Genesis 2 picture of one man and one woman forming one flesh, and suggests that the only alternative to that kind of beautiful sexual intimacy is holy celibacy: being single for the glory of God and the service of God's purposes in the world. It is clear that to be single and sexually unattached is an expression of high human responsibility and high respect for humans everywhere.

Jesus teaches responsible "looking" in the famous "lust" teaching in Matthew 5. We are to sanctify our sexual imagination and be careful not to "look in order to lust." This kind of targeting with the intention of violating a person through fantasy is already the sin of adulterating and trivializing the most sacred part of yourself and the other person. The point Jesus seems to be making is that we must look at every person as valuable, knowing each is a sexual person. We easily celebrate that good gift and leave them to the ecstasy that goes with their own exclusive marriage. This high target, which keeps all of us focused on our own life-long intimacy covenant, means looking ahead toward marriage when we are young and looking back to reconstruct a life-long fidelity for the rest of our lives. This sex-positive focusing of sexual imagination and energy is an invitation to clear and exclusive thinking as the highest respect we can show for everyone. We can imagine intimacy between married partners, the future marriage of our unmarried friends and our own past and future with the exclusive partner of our magical choosing. No one has a higher, more positive view of sex than Jesus.

Divorce: Unspeakable Loss and Pain

Jesus is more impatient with Jewish divorce practices than almost anything else. Read one of his sharp exchanges in Matthew 19 again. One group of Jewish leaders followed the school of Hillel, a leading rabbi. Hillel had taught that Moses' law in Deuteronomy 24, about discovering "some naked thing" about your wife meant "anything displeasing to you." So Jewish men, who were often polygynous, could dismiss wives for any trivial thing at all, much like firing a domestic employee. But the school of Shammai, another great rabbi, taught that only in case of some tragic exposure of past sexual disgrace could a man divorce his wife. So, in Matthew 19, the two groups got Jesus in the crossfire and wanted him to take sides. Instead, he took them back to Genesis, to Creation, and gave them a kindergarten lesson in the meaning of marriage. He hit the crescendo with the warning: "Therefore what God has joined together, let [no one] separate" — a command you will hear at the end of every Christian wedding today.

But watch Jesus, in John 4, deal with a woman who had been married and divorced five times, and who, in this shameful condition, was now living with a man to whom she was not married. Jesus clearly believes that divorce is not the end of hope. He puts her back on the track of abundant life. So Jesus is not simply a purist who shoots the wounded. He believes that anybody in any tragic condition can be salvaged. There is healing and hope for anybody today.

The Ghost of Lost Love

Jesus cautions about establishing a bond with a second partner after having bonded with one's first. His teaching is essentially this: remarriage after divorce [or a break up?] creates grief, and you may take a ghost to bed with your new partner. The rule seems to be that if you divorce, you violate a bond, but that bond is likely to survive and haunt the new marriage. This effect of mixing two bonds is called "adultery" or adulterated bonding. Only when the bond has been killed, mutilated by what Jesus calls "fornication" [also translated "harlotry" or "promiscuity"] can the victim remarry without carrying the ghost of the previous bond into — and thus adulterating — the new sexual relationship.

Read Jesus in Mark 10:11-12. Here Jesus warns both men and women against divorce: "Anyone who divorces his wife and marries another woman commits adultery against her. And if she divorces her husband and marries another man, she commits adultery." Matthew 5:32 and 19:9 add one exception, which if it is present, keeps the adultery ghost from appearing: Anyone who divorces a spouse gets into adultery when they remarry — except when the divorce was a result of fornication — that is, harlotry, promiscuity or what we call sexual addiction.

If you think, *Well I'm not married, so this doesn't apply to me,* think again. If powerful intimate bonding "lives" to haunt the future, it will be important to avoid moving beyond bonding Step 6 until you can slowly move toward Steps 7-8-9 in a realistic and responsible sequence toward a wedding at a fixed calendar date. Remember Step 6 hits "rotation" with Step 7. And a broken bond, even as early as Step 7, 8 or 9, can leave the ghost of a lost love. It is just like Jesus to caution about what one person can do to another. So a rebellious or hard-hearted person can break a relationship or a marriage, but the responsibility falls on that person for "causing the abandoned spouse" to commit adultery by taking a broken heart into another marriage. The victim of abandonment or divorce can take notice, too, that healing time, grief time and slow recovery are essential if they are to enter a new relationship without the ghost haunting their future.

The guidelines here apply equally to breaking up when dating. It is important to pay attention to feelings and attachment and not to jump into a new dating relationship when grief is still heavy from the lost friendship. Otherwise, we mix bonds even though they are at very early stages and are far from becoming sexual. The principle of healing before starting over applies to all of us for a lifetime.

Transformation of Failure and Loss

I pointed you to the famous "woman at the well" story in John 4, to illustrate how Jesus accepted and gave hope to people who had suffered multiple marriages and divorces. In this case, Jesus helped the woman to begin again from where she was. Since women were more likely to be the victims of sexual abuse and divorce in Jesus' day, the clearest examples of his care and affirmation are for such women. In Luke 7:36-50, for example, a "woman who had lived a sinful life" invades a dinner party to bathe Jesus' feet with perfumed water. Jesus takes the occasion to announce her forgiveness and to rebuke the host, who wanted to throw the woman out.

In the opening verses of John 8, a woman who has been "caught in the act of adultery" is dragged to Jesus by Jewish men who want to test Jesus by asking him to pronounce judgment on her. Jesus surprises the men by announcing that only those "without sin" will be permitted to throw stones to execute her. So, again, Jesus is "for" the victims and "against" the proud people with good reputations.

The Apostle Paul reminds the early Christians in Colossians 3:2-15 to remember their own broken past lives:

> Set your minds on things above, not on earthly things. For you died, and your life is now hidden with Christ in God. . . . Put to death, therefore, whatever belongs to your earthly nature: sexual immorality [fornication], impurity, lust, evil desires and greed, which is idolatry. . . . You used to walk in these ways, in the life you once lived. But now you must rid yourselves of all such things as these: anger, rage, malice, slander, and filthy language from your lips. Do not lie to each other, since you have taken off your old self with its practices and have put on the new self, which is being renewed in knowledge in the image of its Creator. . . . Bear with each other and forgive whatever grievances you may have against one another. . . . Let the peace of Christ rule in your hearts . . . ."

The principle is clear: Christians are people who remember their own weakness and failure. They are under reconstruction. So they offer hope and forgiveness to people who fail and who need Jesus' healing grace and hope.

Brides, Grooms, Weddings and Intimacy

When the Bible wants to make its highest and best point, it does it with stories and word pictures of exclusive man-woman relationships that lead to public celebration and sexual intimacy. So, the creation of humans is the peak of the Genesis Creation story, and the detailed version of the human creation in chapter two has the man and woman both formed "bone" and "flesh" from the same Adam. But the plot hits the heavens when the new couple turn out to be spellbound with discovering each other, falling into each others' arms and reuniting the "one flesh!"

So a man and a woman, to this day, enter the best of all possible worlds when they turn away from home and parents and form a new unity, naked and without shame — "one flesh." Together they will, if things go right, form "one flesh" babies who themselves will become women and men in due time. These "bone of my bone, flesh of my flesh" children will then find and form other primary bonds. That story is "as good as it gets."

And when God wants to picture the relationship Diety has with humans, Israel is God's wife, and God is the faithful Husband. The church turns out to be the Body of Christ, the Bride of Christ the Groom. Neither is a "perfect marriage," just as no human marriage is perfect. But God joins with humans to form an eternal, exclusive bond. We are "born into" God's kingdom. We are suckled and nurtured by Mother Church. We may even carry on adolescent "love-hate" battles with Mother Church and with Father God, but we always yearn to "come home" to Jesus, to the Father-Groom and to the Church-Bride and Mother. If we return, it will be with honest repentance and visible eagerness for the reunion.

The ultimate homecoming will also be a wedding. You can read about it in Revelation 19 and 21. Notice in Revelation 18:21-24 the list of things that will never be heard in the evil city, Babylon, again. Among those missing sounds is this: "The voice of bridegroom and bride will never be heard in you again." Weddings are celebrations. Some, unfortunately, may have been preceded by premature intimacy, even "living together." Nevertheless, weddings

Chapter Nine: Take Your Curiosity to the Bible

are public, peak experiences celebrated with the community! But where evil spreads, celebrations fade away. Look at where the celebration of the ages is described in Revelation 19:7 — "The wedding of the Lamb [Jesus] has come, and his bride [the Church] has made herself ready." Notice how the bride is dressed. Notice that those are truly blessed who get an invitation to "the marriage supper" of Jesus and the Church.

Now, turn to Revelation 21 and read from the top. In contrast to Babylon, the evil city, here is Jerusalem, the Holy City — the residence of the true believers, the Church eternal. She is "coming down out of heaven from God, prepared as a bride beautifully dressed for her husband" (21:2). The best news ever announced is this: From this time on God is present, living among the people. "They will be his people, and God himself will be with them and be their God. He will wipe every tear from their eyes" (21:3-4).

All of this final wedding celebration is taking place on the banks of the "river of the water of life, as clear as crystal, flowing from the throne of God and of the Lamb down the middle of the great street of the city" (Revelation 22:1-2). The setting for the "marriage supper of the Lamb" is described in Revelation 22, which contains a final invitation in verse 17. Here it is with plural pronouns to make clear how wide the invitation is: "The Spirit [the Holy Spirit] and the bride say, 'Come!' And let those who hear say, 'Come!' Whoever is thirsty, let them come; and whoever wishes let them take the free gift of the water of life."

Here is the big picture: History begins with a solitary Adam, split into man and woman, who reunite as "one flesh, naked and without shame." And history will end with Jesus, who is called the Second Adam by St. Paul. Jesus, too, was opened at the *pleura* as the tip of a Roman soldier's spear split open his side as he hung on the cross. And Jesus' Bride has been formed out of his opened side. We call her "the Body of Christ: the Church."

So now, at the end of time, the Bride has finally met her Groom at the marriage supper of the Lamb. There both the Bride and the Groom turn out to be Jesus, the Second Adam, split, but being reunited for eternity. That happy wedding is one to which you and I are being invited.

In the meantime, your sexual energy and your yearning for intimacy are among God's most powerful ways of keeping your attention and your affection on the real Wedding. Make your human loving holy and pure, because it is your own personal rehearsal for the real thing, forever. Eternity is far longer than this lifetime; so get ready for the Big Wedding!

So there is the walking tour of what the Bible says about intimacy and sexuality. And this brings us to the point where I must say "Goodbye." I dedicated this book especially to three granddaughters: Lesli, Jami and Heather — my wonderful, beautiful connections to the future.

It is easy to leave these words with you. You will find better words for your children and grandchildren, no doubt. But you have been so kind and supportive to me that I know we absolutely trust each other.

Jami, you showed your faithfulness when you insisted on staying through the night at the medical center, worried that I was spending too many nights with my dying father. I often think of another time you showed your care for me. You were three years old. I was doing some construction work and accidently cut into an artery on the front bone of my lower left leg. As I came toward the house to dress the injury, you watched the blood pumping in a pulsating spray. "Papaw hurt? Fix it?" you asked me. And you toddled into the bathroom behind me while I got my foot into the lavatory to dress the wound and stop the flow of blood. Already you were my loving caregiver.

Heather and Lesli, you recently went down the path of loss twice almost within a year. You laid your Grandmother "Mimi" Luckenbill to rest on Christmas Eve only a year and two weeks before we huddled around Dad's casket. Death is no celebration at all, but you showed your colors of fidelity and care as we went through that loss together. Heather had been the "anchorwoman" interviewing Dad and Mother on video at our tribal Christmas dinner on his last day with us before hospitalization. Then, two weeks later, Lesli, you literally surrounded Mother with your love as you sat glued to her, eyes brimming with tears during our time at the funeral home.

I'm glad I've got the three of you and you've got me — forever, because of Jesus! Carry on well, you new Joy women!

Index:

Abandoning yourself, 38 f.
Abandonment, 80 f.
Abuse, victim of, 11, 79 ff.
   healing for, 80 ff.
   incest, 91 ff.
Acne, 22
Adam, split in Eden, 69
   two become one, 75
Adolescent, 19
Adoption, 16
Adulterating, 104
Arm-to-shoulder, 53
Arm-to-waist, 53 f.
Baal, name for "husband," 101
Birth parents, 16
Bonding, birth, 7
Bonding, pair, 10, 46 ff.
   Desmond Morris' 12 steps, 49 ff.
   foundations for, 52 ff.
   consumating, 57 ff.
   for a lifetime, 58 f.
   sexual, 73 f.
Bonding, crazy, 48 ff.
Brain, female, 75 ff.
Breasts, 21
Brides and grooms, 110 f.
Brothers, 33 ff.
Chromosomes, 70
Co-dependencey, 93 ff.
Coles, Robert, 40
Colossians 3:2-15, 109
Competency, 42
Conception, 68
Corinthians, 2 12:7-10, 75
Crocker, Dr. Max, 12

DNA, mitochondrial, 70
Daniel Boone National Forest, 11
Disaster, another name for "sin," 63
Divorce, 54, 107 f.
Eating disorders, 89
Endorphins, 53
Engagement, 56, 59
Eye-to-Body, 50
Eye-to-Eye, 50
Face-to-face, 60 f.
Family systems, types, 29
Fathers, 29 ff.
    bonding and father absence, 47
Fertility, 20, 68 ff.
Fetus, development, 70
Fornicating, 104
Genesis 1:26-28, 99 100
    2:25, 62
    3, 105
    4:1, 17, 25, 103
    3:15-20, 70
    5: 1-2, 99
    39, 105
Gilligan, Carol, 38 f.
God and the Rhetoric of Sexuality, 99
Hand-to-body, 62
Hand-to-genital, 64
Hand-to-hand, 53
Hand-to-head, 61
Height, 23
    and menstrual period, 23
Hormones, 23
Image of God, 98 ff.
Incest, 91 ff.
Instruments, music, 23
Intimacy, 40 f.
Ish and Ishah, 100, 103
Job 42:15
John 17:20-23, 100
    4, 107

8, 109
Judges 19:20-26
Kissing, intimate, 59
Lafayette High School, 8
Les Miserables, 45
Luke 7:36-50, 109
Lust, 106
Lovers: What ever Happened to Eden? 69
Lying 61
Machisma Female, 83
Macho men, 47 ff.
    Risk-proofing, 64 ff.
Mark 10:11-12, 108
Matthew 1:25, 103
    5, 106
    5:32, 108
    19, 106, 107
Menstruation, 18
Mentors as models, 84
    avoiding "crush," 84
Miscarriage, 68
Morris, Desmond, 49, 57, 60, 62, 63
Monogamy, 52
Mothers, 31 ff.
Mouth-to-breast, 63 f.
Networks, 85 ff.
Ovulation, 19
Pattison, E. Mansell, 86
Privacy, 59
Proverbs 31:1--31, 101
Puberty, 18
Rape, 104 ff.
Recreation, 25
Revelation 21 ff., 111 ff.
Rolling Stone Magazine, 40
Romeo and Juliet, 55
Samuel, 1 1:19, 103
Seduction, 87
Self-esteem, 81, 83 ff.

Self-respect, 81
Sexaholics, 90
Sex and the American Teenager, 40
Sex as "image of God." 98 ff.
Sex differences, 102
Sex in marriage, 42
Sex-negative vs. sex-positive understandings, 98
Sexual addiction, 88
Sexual appetite, 42
Sexual energy, sanctification of, 88 ff.
Sexual experience, premature, 42
Sexual pleasure, 71 f.
Shame, 89
Sisters, 34 ff.
Song of Songs, 50, 106 ff.
Thinking, global, 76
Time, real world vs. intimacy world, 41
Teenager, 18
Teeth, 22
Trible, Phyllis,. 99
Turfland Mall, 15
University of Kentucky Hospital, 7
Voice-to-voice, 51
White Mountain Creamery, 8

CPSIA information can be obtained at www.ICGtesting.com
228148LV00001B/1/P